Polycystic Ovarian Syndrome (PCOS)

A Clinician's Manual

Polycystic Ovarian Syndrome (PCOS)

A Clinician's Manual

Editor

Hemant Deshpande

Professor and Head
Department of Obstetrics and Gynaecology
DY Patil Medical College and Hospital DPU, Pimpri, Pune

Co-editor

Priyanka Dahiya

Assistant Professor
Department of Obstetrics and Gynaecology
Kalpana Chawla Government Medical College, Karnal, Haryana

Foreword

Shirish N Daftary

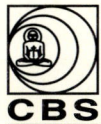

CBS

CBS Publishers & Distributors Pvt Ltd

New Delhi • Bengaluru • Chennai • Kochi • Kolkata • Mumbai

Bhopal • Bhubaneswar • Hyderabad • Jharkhand • Nagpur • Patna • Pune • Uttarakhand • Dhaka (Bangladesh)

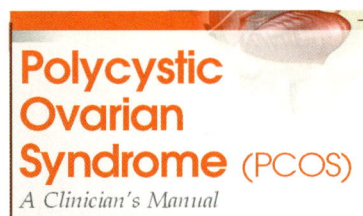

Polycystic Ovarian Syndrome (PCOS)
A Clinician's Manual

ISBN: 978-93-88725-69-9

Published by Satish Kumar Jain and produced by Varun Jain for

CBS Publishers & Distributors Pvt Ltd
4819/XI Prahlad Street, 24 Ansari Road, Daryaganj, New Delhi 110 002
Ph: 23289259, 23266861, 23266867   Fax: 011-23243014   Website: www.cbspd.com
e-mail: delhi@cbspd.com; cbspubs@airtelmail.in

Corporate Office: 204 FIE, Industrial Area, Patparganj, Delhi 110 092
Ph: 4934 4934   Fax: 4934 4935   e-mail: publishing@cbspd.com; publicity@cbspd.com

Branches

- **Bengaluru:** Seema House 2975, 17th Cross, K.R. Road,
  Banasankari 2nd Stage, Bengaluru 560 070, Karnataka
  Ph: +91-80-26771678/79   Fax: +91-80-26771680   e-mail: bangalore@cbspd.com
- **Chennai:** 7, Subbaraya Street, Shenoy Nagar, Chennai 600 030, Tamil Nadu
  Ph: +91-44-26260666, 26208620   Fax: +91-44-42032115   e-mail: chennai@cbspd.com
- **Kochi:** 42/1325, 1326, Power House Road, Opp KSEB Power House, Ernakulam 682 018, Kochi, Kerala
  Ph: +91-484-4059061-65   Fax: +91-484-4059065   e-mail: kochi@cbspd.com
- **Kolkata:** No. 6/B, Ground Floor, Rameswar Shaw Road, Kolkata-700014 (West Bengal), India
  Ph: +91-33-2289-1126, 2289-1127, 2289-1128   e-mail: kolkata@cbspd.com
- **Mumbai:** 83-C, Dr E Moses Road, Worli, Mumbai-400018, Maharashtra
  Ph: +91-22-24902340/41   Fax: +91-22-24902342   e-mail: mumbai@cbspd.com

Representatives

- Bhopal   0-8319310552
- Jharkhand   0-9811541605
- Pune   0-9623451994
- Bhubaneswar 0-9911037372
- Nagpur   0-9421945513
- Uttarakhand 0-9716462459
- Hyderabad   0-9885175004
- Patna   0-9334159340
- Dhaka (Bangladesh) 01912-003485

Printed at: HT Media Ltd., Greater Noida, UP, India

to

Sadguru Shri Raghvendra Swami Ji

Foreword

It gives me immense pleasure to thank the editors—Dr Hemant Deshpande and Dr Priyanka Dahiya for compiling this monogram entitled *Polycystic Ovarian Syndrome (PCOS)*.

PCOS is a heterogenous, multisystem endocrinopathy affecting women in the reproductive age with the ovarian expression clinically presenting as menstrual disturbances, anovulatory infertility and a plethora of metabolic manifestations such as obesity, impaired glucose tolerance and hyperandrogenism presenting as hirsutism and acne. These women in the younger age group often seek the advice of the gynaecologist for their problem of menstrual irregularity or infertility. It is, therefore, incumbent on our fraternity to comprehend the wider implications of this syndrome and present a holistic approach in its management. PCOS, left untreated may be the harbinger of future diseases like cardiovascular disease, diabetes and endometrial cancer. Much progress has been achieved in recognition and management of PCOS since its first recognition by Stein and Leventhal in 1935. Increased clinical awareness, imaging facilities and hormone assays have contributed immensely towards a better understanding of the disease and its management. There has been immense evolvement in its management since Stein - Leventhal first suggested 'wedge resection' to the modern times of *in vitro* maturation and oocyte cryopreservation. PCOS is a multidimensional entity. There is so much to look at that one gets lost in a maze. Many disciplines are now involved in investigation of the syndrome from endocrinologists, metabolic experts, dermatologists and cosmetologists.

An attempt has been made to present a plethora of knowledge by experts in this field in a well dispensed and simplified form as a brief ready reckoner. The book truly unveils the origins, epigenetics, autoimmunity and pathophysiology aspects of PCOS. Besides these, it thoroughly deals with the metabolic aspects and its long-term implications contributing to pregnancy complications, and impact on adolescent health and concerns.

This monograph also covers extensively the pharmacological and surgical management PCOS as well as the role of adjuvant therapies.

I am impressed with the attempt by the editors to bring on the same page various distinguished faculty members from all over India. They have done a commendable job of the tasks assigned to them. They have left no stone unturned to truly unveil the mysteries of PCOS. Each chapter is supported by an up-to-date list of references, and the comprehensive index covers all the useful topics.

The editors of this book, Dr Hemant Deshpande and Dr Priyanka Dahiya have accomplished a herculean task and deserve our heartiest congratulations. This comprehensive monogram will surely encourage our younger colleagues to design future research until we finally have all the answers.

Shirish N Daftary

Former Professor of Obstetrics and Gynaecology, Seth GS Medical College
Former Dean and Emeritus Professor, Nowrosji Wadia Maternity Hospital
Former President, FOGSI
Editor of several publications

Preface

PCOS constitutes a bulk (80%) of cases of anovulatory infertility. Research done in recent years has facilitated a greater understanding of the complex genetic, biochemical, metabolic factors involved in the etiopathogenesis of PCOS. The book titled *Polycystic Ovarian Syndrome (PCOS)* presents an invaluable tool for those with interest in reproductive medicine as well as those in field of infertility.

Not only does this ailment have a diverse presentation, it also mutates its intensity and progress in an individual over time. A greater incidence and understanding about the origin of PCOS, its pathophysiology and genetics have spawned a lot of publications and research in this domain.

This attempt is unique as it provides a comprehensive and yet concise review of the environmental factors and lifestyle choices as important cofactors in the genesis of this condition and its impact on fertility. Special emphasis has been laid on the origin and role of autoimmunity in PCOS, complete etiopathogenesis, long-term implications, associated complications during pregnancy, and medical and surgical management. It offers a comprehensive review of contemporary protocols in the both diagnosis and treatment of female infertility.

In writing this book, I have many people to whom I owe a great deal. A heartfelt thanks to all my contributors.

Written in clear concise and readable style, this volume allows the reader to obtain rapid answers to this challenging medical issues. It also covers the latest research in female infertility.

I hope that the effort has all been worthwhile and that this book will be of value to students and clinicians involved in management of infertility.

We assure you to unravel mystery associated with PCOS.......

Hemant Deshpande

Priyanka Dahiya

Acknowledgements

The economic and societal burden of infertility is high and increasing with time. Today PCOS is recognized in women as single most common cause of androgen excess, one of the most frequent causes of infertility and possibly the most common hormonal abnormality.

In past two decades, we also begun to understand the association of PCOS with metabolic abnormalities, including insulin resistance, hyperinsulinemia and glucose intolerance. Hippocrates, in around 400 BC, described two cases of women with excess hair growth and whose menses ceased. Only in last century have the ovaries been recognized as hormonal origin of these symptoms.

PCOS excites immense interest and debate. Not only may the presentation vary, but also the nature of condition in an individual may change over time. As we have begun to understand more about the origins of PCOS, its pathophysiology and genetics, we have seen an exponential rise in the number of publications in this exciting area of medicine. The management of PCOS is not without controversy—from making diagnosis to the appropriate forms of therapy, and there are some differences around the world. This book provides its readers, with an up-to-date accessible text of a medical condition whose prevalence is going to increase in the coming years.

I would like to thank all my contributors for neatly and timely submission of articles for this book.

I would like to thank my wife Dr Anjali Deshpande for bearing with me and giving her time in making this book.

I will put on record my appreciation to Mr Ramesh Krishnamachari, Mr YN Arjuna and Ms Ritu Chawla of CBS Publication for assisting in the editorial process efficiently and promptly.

Hemant Deshpande

List of Contributors

Astha Shrivastava
Assistant Professor
Dept of Obstetrics and Gynaecology
Lady Hardinge Medical College, New Delhi

Abha Singh
Director, Professor and Head
Department of Obstetrics and Gynaecology
Lady Hardinge Medical College, New Delhi

Amarjeet Kaur
Sr Resident
Department of Obstetrics and Gynaecology
GMC, Amritsar

Amey Chugh
Senior Resident
Department of Obstetrics and Gynaecology
DY Patil Medical College and Hospital, Pune

Amrita Chaurasia
Professor and Head
Department of Obstetrics and Gynaecology
MLN Medical College, Allahabad

Anjali Deshpande
Pathologist
DY Patil Medical College and Hospital, Pune

Anjali Gupta
Professor
Department of Obstetrics and Gynaecology
Pt BD Sharma PGIMS, Rohtak, Haryana

Arindam Halder
Assistant Professor
Department of Obstetrics and Gynaecology
Cittaranjan Seva Sadan, Kolkata

Ashok Kumar
Director Professor
Department of Obstetrics and Gynaecology
Maulana Azad Medical College and Lok Nayak
Hospital, New Delhi

B Ramesh
Laparoscopic Surgeon and Director
Altius Hospital, Bengaluru

Chandrakant Madkar
Professor
Department of Obstetrics and Gynaecology
DY Patil Medical College and Hospital, Pune

Divya KV
Resident
Department of Obstetrics and Gynaecology
Maulana Azad Medical College and Lok Nayak
Hospital, New Delhi

Garima Sharma
Consultant IVF Specialist
EVA Care Fertility Centre, Mumbai

Himadri Bal
Professor
Department of Obstetrics and Gynaecology
DY Patil Medical College and Hospital, Pune

Hiralal Konar
Professor
Agartala Government Medical College, Agartala
Tripura

Hemant Deshpande
Professor and Head
Department of Obstetrics and Gynaecology
DY Patil Medical College and Hospital, Pune

Jai Bhagwan Sharma
Professor
Department of Obstetrics and Gynaecology
AIIMS, New Delhi

Kiran Pandey
Professor and Head
Department of Obstetrics and Gynaecology
GSVM Medical College, Kanpur

Madhukar Shinde
Associate Professor
Department of Obstetrics and Gynaecology
DY Patil Medical College, Pune

Monica Gupta
Fellow Reproductive Medicine
Department of Obstetrics and Gynaecology
AIIMS, New Delhi

Munjal Pandya
Assistant Professor
Department of Obstetrics and Gynaecology
AMC MET Medical College and Sheth LG Hospital
Ahmedabad

Pankaj Desai
Professor and Head of Unit
Department of Obstetrics and Gynaecology
VRS Medical College and SSG Hospital, Baroda

Pavika Lal
Assistant Professor
Department of Obstetrics and Gynaecology
GSVM Medical College, Kanpur

Picklu Chaudhuri
Professor
Department of Obstetrics and Gynaecology
Rampurhat Medical College, Birbhum, West Bengal

Priyanka Dahiya
Assistant Professor
Department of Obstetrics and Gynaecology
Kalpana Chawla Government Medical College, Karnal

Rajendra Shitole
Assistant Professor
Department of Obstetrics and Gynaecology
DY Patil Medical College and Hospital, Pune

Ratnakant Talukdar
Professor and Head
Department of Obstetrics and Gynaecology
Guwahati Medical College, Guwahati

Richa Kansal
Professor and Head
Department of Obstetrics and Gynaecology
Kalpana Chawla Government Medical College, Karnal

Savita Rani Singhal
Professor
Department of Obstetrics and Gynaecology
Pt. BD Sharma PGIMS, Rohtak, Haryana

Shipra Kunwar
Professor and Head
Department of Obstetrics and Gynaecology
Ira Medical College, Lucknow

Smiti Nanda
Professor and Head
Department of Obstetrics and Gynaecology
Pt. BD Sharma PGIMS, Rohtak, Haryana

Suman Mittal
Professor
Department of Obstetrics and Gynaecology
SMS Medical College, Jaipur

Sukesh Kumar Kathpalia
Professor
Department of Obstetrics and Gynaecology
DY Patil Medical College and Hospital, Pune

Suyajna D Joshi
Ex-Professor and HOD
Department of Obstetrics and Gynaecology
VIMS, Bellary, Karnatka

Sujata Sharma
Professor and Head
Department of Obstetrics and Gynaecology
Govt. Medical College, Amritsar

Shashwat Jani
Assistant Professor
Department of Obstetrics and Gynaecology
Smt NHL Municipal Medical College, Ahmedabad

Tapan Shah
Assistant Professor
Department of General Surgery
Smt NHL Municipal Medical College, Ahmedabad

Umesh Sable
Assistant Professor
Department of Obstetrics and Gynaecology
DY Patil Medical College and Hospital, Pune

Unmesh S Santpur
Professor
Department of Obstetrics and Gynaecology
Maharishi Markandeshwar Institue of Medical Sciences
and Research
Mullana, Ambala

Vandana Rani
Assistant Professor
Department of Obstetrics and Gynaecology
Pt BD Sharma PGIMS, Rohtak, Haryana

Contents

Unveiling the Origin of PCOS

Amrita Chaurasia

Polycystic ovary syndrome (PCOS) is a widespread reproductive disorder that encompasses many associated health conditions and has an impact on various metabolic processes. Despite increasing incidence of PCOS, there are several aspects that remain ambiguous. Currently, there is no consensus on the origin of PCOS. In this review; the past, the current and the possible future perspectives regarding the origin of PCOS will be discussed. A better insight into the early origins and natural history of hyperinsulinemic androgen excess may sharpen the perspective of PCOS prevention.

ANCIENT MEDICAL RECORDS

PCOS has an ancient genetic stamp and references to the syndrome that go back as far as the ancient Egyptian papyri and shown up repeatedly in ancient Greek and Hebrew literatures as well as the medieval and Renaissance periods. These ancient literatures have described PCOS like phenotype in their own peculiar ways.[1]

Here are some of the descriptions from these literatures:

"But those women whose menstruation is less than three days or is meagre, are robust, with a healthy complexion and a masculine appearance; yet they are not concerned about bearing children nor do they become pregnant."

"Sometimes it is also natural not to menstruate at all... It is natural too in persons whose bodies are of a masculine type... we observe that the majority of those not menstruating are rather robust, like mannish and sterile women."

"...there are women whose skin is dry and hard, and whose nature resembles the nature of a man. However, if any woman's nature tends to be transformed to the nature of a man, this does not arise from medications, but is caused by heavy menstrual activity."

"Many women, when their flowers or tearmes be stopped, degenerate after a manner into a certain manly nature, whence they are called Viragines, that is to stay stout, or manly women; therefore their voice is loud and bigge, like unto a mans, and they become bearded."[1]

These statements made over a period of more than two millennia describing a combination of symptoms, including menstrual irregularity, masculine habitus, subfertility and obesity are suggestive of PCOS existence during ancient times and was sufficiently common too, to merit description.[2]

Our ancestors described it as a 'fertility problem', but at the same time surprisingly it was also considered a 'survival factor'. Though they were unable to explain the reason, people with insulin resistance survived better when food was hard to get and everyone had to work hard physically to create shelter and stay safe.[3] Now we also understand that PCOS is associated with insulin resistance that actually imparts a relative 'fuel efficiency'; an advantage in times of food scarcity.

In present scenario as food is easily available and one does not have to struggle hard physically to get it; the obesity, diabetes, heart disease and other PCOS-related complications have no more left PCOS as a 'survival factor'!

EVOLVING RESEARCHES TO KNOW THE ORIGIN OF PCOS

The Concept of 'Prenatal Androgen Excess'

Way back in 1982, Goy and Robinson experimented on animal models; the rhesus monkey and sheep and showed that animals exposed prenatally to an exogenous excess of androgens had ambiguous genitalia, fetal growth restraint, virilized behavior and emergence of PCOS-like phenotype including hyper-insulinemic androgen excess, polycystic ovaries, elevated levels of circulating LH, dyslipidemia, visceral adiposity, and reduced ovulation rate particularly in overweight adults.[4–6] With such consistent evidences, the concept of 'prenatal androgen excess' came into view. In year 1989, Hickey *et al* tested the 'prenatal androgen excess' hypothesis for the first time in humans.[7] They performed a longitudinal study of 244 unselected girls recruited prenatally along with their mothers to test maternal androgenemia (through pregnancy) and fetal androgenemia (at birth) into the Raine cohort; initiated by John Newnham and followed them till the age approximately 15 years to be diagnosed with PCOS by NIH or Rotterdam criteria. The authors concluded that their findings did not support the hypothesis of 'prenatal androgen excess'.

However, for many reasons, it was too premature to abandon this hypothesis completely with the possible probability of missing a brief window of maternal or fetal androgen excess by the researchers. Additionally, the applied PCOS definitions might not be valid for 15-yr-old adolescents and thus may have been misleading.

Later in years 1998 and 2002, studies by Padmanabhan and co-workers in sheep and by Abbott and colleagues in the rhesus

monkey again affirmed that animals exposed to high levels of androgen *in utero* (by giving very large doses of androgen to the mothers) developed as adults with disrupted ovarian cycles, abnormalities of early follicle development, metabolic abnormalities including insulin resistance and impaired glucose tolerance, mimicking PCOS.[3, 5–6, 8–12] Thus, the hypothesis of androgen programming *in utero* or during postnatal development as an important aspect in the origin of PCOS again gained currency.

However, doubts on the plausibility of this hypothesis persisted and many questions remained unanswered. Because the fetus is buffered against maternal androgen excess in human pregnancy due to the twin barriers of high levels of SHBG and placental aromatase activity, androgen of mother is hard to cross the placenta unless compromised placental function, such as placental aromatase deficiency, stress or inadequate diet is there.

So the question arose, from where does the excess fetal androgen come from and when and how are its effects exerted? And secondly, why PCOS women do not have ambiguous genitals?

The explained hypothesis says that it is not the maternal androgen excess that affects the fetus but the presence of genetically predisposed fetal ovaries or adrenal cortex or both hypersecrete androgens during fetal life or during infancy or during reawakening of the hypothalamic-pituitary-gonadal axis during puberty[13–16] causing hyperandrogenemia and their consequences.

Prenatal androgens produced during fetal organ differentiation are also described as potent gene transcription factors that permanently enhance gene expression (including increased serine phosphorylation of the cAMP response element) related to insulin resistance and hyperinsulinemia.[17] A recent study by Abbott and others done in 2011 in the rhesus monkey also suggested that developmental programming by prenatal androgen exposure involves epigenetic regulation.[18] It is, therefore, feasible that fetal androgen excess in human females simultaneously reprograms multiple organ systems that will later manifest the heterogeneous phenotype of PCOS.

One of the recent publications that looked in detail at both reproductive and metabolic consequences of androgen excess in rodent model has shown the findings of enlarged adipocytes and decreased serum levels of adiponectin similar to those in women with PCOS, depicting the relationship between excess androgen, obesity and metabolic dysfunction.[19–21]

Virilization of female genitalia, as a result of excess fetal androgen, does not occur in women with PCOS. Prenatal androgen excess does not cause virilization in humans because it has been found to exert subtle but permanent effects on female physiology only.[16, 22]

It has also been shown that cultured human theca cells from polycystic ovaries produce 20 times more androstenedione than similar cells from normal ovaries.[23] The exaggerated ovarian androgen response to exogenous human chorionic gonadotropin (hCG) or endogenous gonadotropins due to increased mRNA expression for many steroidogenic enzymes.[24–27] The genes encoding steroidogenic enzyme were identified in the promoter region of CYP11a.[28] But at the same time, it is unlikely to be the exclusive cause of PCOS because the complex PCOS phenotype seems hard to believe to be due to a single gene defect only.

Prenatally androgenized rhesus monkeys and ewes also have abnormal LH secretions; that is described to be due to permanently diminished hormonal negative feedback on the hypothalamic–pituitary axis during gestation as well as post-puberty. During intra-uterine life, this fetal pituitary LH individually or along with placental hCG and genes regulating folliculogenesis and steroidogenesis further result in fetal ovarian hyperandrogenemia leading to prenatal androgen excess and its potential consequences.

In post-pubertal period, abnormally raised LH predisposes the girl to adiposity (basically central) exaggerating insulin resistance. The resultant hyperinsulinemia synergistically interacts with LH hypersecretion to alter ovarian steroidogenesis, premature arrest of follicle development, anovulation and polycystic ovaries.

The similarity of reproductive and metabolic phenotype between prenatally androgenized sheep, or monkeys, and women with PCOS provides strong supportive evidence for intra-uterine developmental programming being important in the etiology of PCOS.

The Concept of 'Adipose Tissue Expendability'

The 'adipose tissue expendability' hypothesis, recently proposed by Virtue and Vidal-Puig, explains the apparent paradox that insulin resistance may occur not only in obese but also when there is a deficit of adipose tissue.[8, 29] The concept says that metabolic health is maintained till the subcutaneous adipose depot can accommodate the caloric supply safely without causing lipotoxicity. When the subcutaneous adipose tissue has a limited capacity to increase its mass safely like in non-obese PCOS women, the adipocytes become overfilled even with the slight fat excess and a lipotoxic state along with dyslipidemia occurs. Lipid starts getting deposited in non-adipose organs such as liver, muscle, or pancreas adversely affecting the metabolism, most notably the insulin action. The concept thus implies that there is an individual set point of subcutaneous lipid storage beyond which lipotoxicity occurs and explains sporadic development of PCOS in women either non-obese or obese.

In obese women with PCOS, obesity exhausts the normal capacity to store subcutaneous fat leading to lipotoxicity and its metabolic complications including hyperinsulinemia, androgen excess, and thus PCOS.[30] Non-obese women who have PCOS may have lesser subcutaneous fat storage capacity putting them under risk of lipotoxicity and insulin resistance. Such non-obese adolescents with PCOS respond better to insulin sensitizers like metformin, pioglitazone, or their combination with flutamide without the need of lowering body weight.[6,10,12] Adipose tissue expendability concept of PCOS thus emphasizes individually tailored therapeutic weight loss with an aim to reduce the weight until a woman's maximal fuel storage capacity remains there.

Girls with a history of low birth weight and precocious pubarche (appearance of pubic hair before age 8 year) have been found to be at risk for developing hyperinsulinemic androgen excess.[3,11] Accordingly, an increment of weight gain in early life may be among one of the effective approaches to prevent PCOS in later life. Accelerated expansion of adipose tissue before birth and in early infancy has been described to confer protection against developing PCOS in adulthood, perhaps by augmenting the recruitment of subcutaneous adipocytes and hence adequate capacity to store fat.[18] Thus prepubertal and pubertal metformin therapy in girls, who were low birth weight and developing precocious puberty, seems rationale to prevent the development of PCOS during adolescence.[31] But advocation of such preventive insulin sensitizer therapies needs much more robust evidence.

The adipose tissue expendability hypothesis also partly explains the ethnic variation of PCOS and the rationale of how better capacity to store subcutaneous fat make the women escape from developing hyperinsulinemia and androgen excess. Caucasian background confers more subcutaneous capacity for fat storage than a South Asian or Far Eastern origin and so more avoidance of developing PCOS. Indian, Chinese, and Japanese women tend to develop hyperinsulinemic androgen excess and polycystic ovaries at being comparatively lesser over-

weight than Caucasian women because of ethnically reduced fat storage capacity. More occurrence of PCOS in countries like India, Pakistan, and Bangladesh, where still about one-fourth of the girls have a birth weight below 2.5 kg again can also be explained by this hypothesis.

The linkage between the two hypothesis of origin of PCOS, *The concept of 'prenatal androgen excess' and The concept of 'adipose tissue expendability'*, seems to exist as testosterone and dihydrotestosterone are known potent inhibitors of adipogenic differentiation of preadipocytes into adipocytes,[13] the females exposed to prenatal androgen excess could have reduced subcutaneous adipogenesis and adipocytes with reduced capacity of subcutaneous fat deposition and thus increased risk of lipotoxicity and related metabolic consequences and PCOS.

The 'Concept of Genetic Association'

The physiological studies fail to tell us whether it is the elevated androgen levels that lead to insulin resistance or insulin resistance leads to hyperandrogenism and polycystic ovarian morphology or they are a result of increased hypothalamic GnRH secretion drives. A better insight into the epigenetics will probably sharpen the perspective of PCOS origin, identification of at-risk girls, prevention and individualization of therapy.

An increasing number of publications infer that genetics is the primary factor of this disease and associated metabolic complications that is further imposed by its sporadic occurrence among both male and female first-degree relatives of women with PCOS. This genetic association theory also explains that positive family history appears to put the women at risk for the development of PCOS and environmental factors alter the clinical and biochemical parameters in only those with genetic predispositions for PCOS.

The clear genetics of PCOS remains unknown but recent studies indicate this multipronged disease to be a complex familial trait where several genes combine with environmental and genetic factors to provoke PCOS phenotype.[32]

Till now, researchers had believed excess testosterone production by the ovary during prenatal period, infancy and adolescent period as major initial culprit in developing PCOS and hyperinsulinemia. Hyperinsulinemia and hyperandrogenemia have also been said to be highly heritable parameters transmitted probably as mendelian autosomal dominant or X-linked traits, but the genetic studies have not as yet concluded the pattern of heredity.[33–35]

The current genetic studies are now shifting the focus more on polygenic disturbances especially related to gonadotropin alterations, androgen hypersecretions and insulin resistance explaining the gonadotropin alterations as well.

GWAS (Genome Wide Association Studies) are now new avenues in PCOS researches and at the forefront of genetic technologies shedding light on the biological pathways underlying complex disorders.[36] Till date, a few GWAS have been published in the field of PCOS, which have been done in Han Chinese women, Korean women and North European women. The first GWAS in Chinese women identified three novel PCOS susceptibility loci, namely, 2p16.3, 2p21, and 9q33.3, which mapped to the genomic areas of three genes LHCGR, THADA, and DENND1A, respectively.[37] A second GWAS in a larger sample of Han Chinese women confirmed the previously identified loci and revealed association of eight new loci which corresponded to genomic regions, thus total eleven genetic loci were found to be involved in insulin signaling, hormonal functions, folliculogenesis, and T2DM-associated genes in addition to calcium signaling and endocytosis and associated hormonal and metabolic disturbances with PCOS. A third GWAS performed in Korean population identified GYS2 to be significantly associated only with the obese subgroup of PCOS women. Dr Andrea Dunaif's team genotyped nearly 700,000 genetic markers from nearly 9,000 women from the US and Europe, and have identified two new genetic susceptibility regions that appeared to be unique to European women.[38]

Ethnicity has influenced over the diverse phenotype in PCOS. Louwers' group study concluded the existence of a common genetic risk profile for PCOS across these populations with slightly definite variations. Further resequencing and fine-mapping of the loci identified in Chinese GWAS were carried out to verify associations in Caucasian populations with PCOS. These replication studies have established the association of DENND1A variants with PCOS susceptibility, hyperandrogenism and unfavorable lipid profiles in affected women. On discovery of a signal for the FSH gene by Dr Andrea Dunaif, which suggested that along with LH and FSH how it acts on the ovary or how it is secreted, is very important in the development of PCOS. This is a new way of thinking about the biology of PCOS.[37, 38]

To conclude, the etiology of polycystic ovary syndrome (PCOS) has been difficult to determine because its features are heterogeneous, and thus its origin also to be heterogeneous. While the GWAS discoveries are throwing new lights on its origin and pathogenesis, they must be confirmed by candidate gene-based replication studies in various ethnic populations. There is no denying that this fast paced field offers immense potential to pinpoint genes affecting the biological processes involved in etiology of multidimensional polygenic disorders like PCOS. Next Dunaif's team have planned to investigate the genomes of women from African ancestry, in order to get better insight into the shared genetic basis for PCOS in that population too. The next years will be very exciting times as groups from around the world come together to further elucidate the genetic origins of PCOS in different continents.

CONCLUSION

While developmental determinants of PCOS altogether remain yet to be determined, it is difficult to view PCOS as purely developmental or resulting only from intrauterine exposures of androgens or simply as an adaptation gone astray. Unveiling the origin of PCOS till now has revealed multiple unveiled factors yet to be revealed and recognized. These unveiled factors lay down many possible fields of researches in the future perspectives of the syndrome.

REFERENCES

1. Early Origins of Polycystic Ovary Syndrome: Hypotheses May Change without Notice: Francis de Zegher Lourdes Ibaìnþez. *The Journal of Clinical Endocrinology and Metabolism*, Volume 94, Issue 10, 1 October 2009, Pages 3682–3685.

2. Azziz Ricardo, Daniel A Dumesic, Mark O Goodarzi. Polycystic ovary syndrome: An ancient disorder?; 2011; 95(5): 1544–48.

3. Abbott DH, Dumesic DA, Eisner JR, Colman RJ, Kemnitz JW. Insights into the development of polycystic ovary syndrome (PCOS) from studies of prenatally androgenized female rhesus monkeys. Trends Endocrinol Metab 1998; 9:62–67.

4. Goy RW, Robinson JA. Insulin resistance and the polycystic ovary syndrome: mechanism and implications for pathogenesis. Endocr Rev 1982; 18: 774–800.

5. Steckler T, Manikkam M, Inskeep EK, Padmanabhan V. Developmental programming: follicular persistence in prenatal testosterone-treated sheep is not programmed by androgenic actions of testosterone. Endocrinology 2007; 148:3532–40.

6. Padmanabhan V, Veiga-Lopez A. Developmental origin of reproductive and metabolic dysfunctions: androgenic versus estrogenic reprogramming. Semin Reprod Med 2011; 29:173–186.

7. Hickey M, Sloboda DM, Atkinson HC, Doherty DA, Franks S, Norman RJ, Newnham JP, Hart R. Developmental programming: excess weight gain amplifies the effects of prenatal testosterone excess on reproductive cyclicity—implication to PCOS. Endocrinology 2009; 150:1456–65.

8. Birch RA, Padmanabhan V, Foster DL, Unsworth WP, Robinson JE. Prenatal programming of reproductive neuroendocrine function: fetal androgen exposure produces progressive disruption of reproductive cycles in sheep. Endocrinology 2003; 144:1426–1434.

9. Steckler T, Wang J, Bartol FF, Roy SK, Padmanabhan V. Fetal programming: prenatal testosterone treatment causes intrauterine growth retardation, reduces ovarian reserve and increases ovarian follicular recruitment. Endocrinology 2005; 146:3185–3193.

10. Veiga-Lopez A, Steckler TL, Abbott DH, Welch KB, MohanKumar PS, Phillips DJ, Refsal K, Padmanabhan V. Developmental programming: impact of excess prenatal testosterone on intrauterine fetal endocrine milieu and growth in sheep. Biol Reprod 2011; 84:87–96.

11. Abbott DH, Tarantal AF, Dumesic DA. Fetal, infant, adolescent and adult phenotypes of polycystic ovary syndrome in prenatally androgenized female rhesus monkeys. Am J Primatol 2009; 71:776–784.

12. Forsdike RA, Hardy K, Bull L, Stark J, Webber LJ, Stubbs S, Robinson JE, Franks S. Disordered follicle development in ovaries of prenatally androgenized ewes. J Endocrinol 2007; 192:421–428.

13. Cole B, Hensinger K, Maciel GA, Chang RJ, Erickson GF. Human fetal ovary development involves the spatiotemporal expression of p450c17 protein. J Clin Endocrinol Metab 2006; 91:3654–3661.

14. Barbieri RL, Saltzman DH, Torday JS, Randall RW, Frigoletto FD and Ryan KJ. Elevated concentrations of the beta-subunit of human chorionic gonadotropin and testosterone in the amniotic fluid of gestations of diabetic mothers. American Journal of Obstetrics and Gynecology 1986; 154:1039–1043.

15. Beck-Peccoz P, Padmanabhan V, Baggiani AM, Cortelazzi D, Buscaglia M, Medri G, Marconi AM, PardiG and Beitins IZ. Maturation of hypothalamic–pituitary–gonadal function in normal human fetuses: circulating levels of gonadotropins, their common alpha-subunit and free testosterone, and discrepancy between immunological and biological activities of circulating follicle stimulating hormone. Journal

of Clinical Endocrinology and Metabolism 1991; 73:525–532.

16. Barnes RB, Rosenfield RL, Ehrmann DA, Cara JF, Cutler L, Levitsky LL and Rosenthal IM. Ovarian hyperandrogenism as a result of congenital adrenal virilizing disorders: evidence for perinatal masculinization of neuroendocrine function in women. Journal of Clinical Endocrinology and Metabolism 1994; 79:1328–1333.

17. Auger AP, Hexter DP and McCarthy MM. Sex difference in the phosphorylation of cAMP response element binding protein (CREB) in neonatal rat brain. Brain Research 2001; 890:110–117.

18. Xu N, Kwon S, Abbott DH, Geller DH, Dumesic DA, Azziz R, Guo X, Goodarzi MO. Epigenetic mechanism underlying the development of polycystic ovary syndrome (PCOS)-like phenotypes in prenatally androgenized rhesus monkeys. PLoS One 2011; 6:e27286.

19. Rodent models for human polycystic ovary syndrome. Biol Reprod February 2012; 10.1095/biolreprod. 111.097808.

20. Barber TM, Hazell M, Christodoulides C, Golding SJ, Alvey C, Burling K, Vidal-Puig A, Groome NP, Wass JA, Franks S, McCarthy MI. Serum levels of retinol-binding protein 4 and adiponectin in women with polycystic ovary syndrome: associations with visceral fat but no evidence for fat mass-independent effects on pathogenesis in this condition. J Clin Endocrinol Metab 2008; 93:2859–2865.

21. Manneräs-Holm L, Leonhardt H, Kullberg J, Jennische E, Odén A, Holm G, Hellström M, Lönn L, Olivecrona G, Stener-Victorin E, LönnM. Adipose tissue has aberrant morphology and function in PCOS: enlarged adipocytes and low serum adiponectin, but not circulating sex steroids, are strongly associated with insulin resistance. J Clin Endocrinol Metab 2011; 96:E304 –E311

22. Herman RA, Jones B, Mann DR and Wallen K. Timing of prenatal androgen exposure: anatomical and endocrine effects on juvenile male and female rhesus monkeys. Hormones and Behavior 2000; 38:52–66.

23. Gilling-Smith C, Willis DS, Beard RW and Franks S. Hypersecretion of androstenedione by isolated theca cells from polycystic ovaries. Journal of Clinical Endocrinology and Metabolism 1994; 79:1158–1165.

24. Gilling-Smith C, Story H, RogersV and Franks S. Evidence for a primary abnormality of thecal

cell steroidogenesis in the polycystic ovary syndrome. Clinical Endocrinology 1997; 47:93–99.

25. Ehrmann DA, Barnes RB and Rosenfield RL. Polycystic ovary syndrome as a form of functional ovarian hyperandrogenism due to dysregulation of androgen secretion. Endocrine Reviews 1995; 16: 322–353.

26. White DW, Leigh A, Wilson C, Donaldson A and Franks S. Gonadotrophin and gonadal steroid response to a single dose of a long-acting agonist of gonadotrophin-releasing hormone in ovulatory and anovulatory women with poly-cystic ovary syndrome. Clinical Endocrinology 1995; 42:475–481.

27. Wickenheisser JK, Quinn PG, Nelson VL, Legro RS, Strauss JF and McAllister JM. Differential activity of the cytochrome P450 17 alpha-hydroxylase and steroidogenic acute regulatory protein gene promoters in normal and polycystic ovary syndrome theca cells. Journal of Clinical Endocrinology and Metabolism 2000; 85:2304–2311.

28. Waterworth DM, Bennett ST, Gharani N, McCarthy M, Hague S, Batty S, Conway GS, White DW, Todd JA, Franks S and Williamson R. Linkage and association of insulin gene VNTR regulatory polymorphism with polycystic ovary syndrome. Lancet 1997; 349:986–990.

29. Maciel GA, Baracat EC, Benda JA, Markham SM, Hensinger K, Chang RJ, Erickson GF. Stockpiling of transitional and classic primary follicles in ovaries of women with polycystic ovary syndrome. J Clin Endocrinol Metab 2004; 89:5321–5327.

30. Hogg K, Wood C, McNeilly AS, Duncan WC. The in utero programming effect of increased maternal androgens and a direct fetal intervention on liver and metabolic function in adult sheep. PLoS One 2011; 6:e24877.

31. Webber LJ, Stubbs S, Stark J, Trew GH, Margara R, Hardy K, Franks S. Formation and early development of follicles in the polycystic ovary. Lancet 2003; 362:1017–1021.

32. Mortensen M, Ehrmann DA, Littlejohn E, Rosenfield RL. Clinical expression of polycystic ovary syndrome in adolescent girls. Fertil Steril 2009; 86(Suppl 1):S6.

33. Moran LJ, Pasquali R, Teede HJ, Hoeger KM, Norman RJ. Modulation of gonadotropin-releasing hormone pulse generator sensitivity to progesterone inhibition in hyperandrogenic adolescent girls—implications for regulation of

pubertal maturation. J Clin Endocrinol Metab 3 December 2008; 94:2360–2366.

34. Fertil Steril Vantyghem MC, Vincent-Desplanques D, Defrance-Faivre F, Capeau J, Fermon C, Valat AS, Lascols O, Hecart AC, Pigny P, Delemer B, Vigouroux C, Wemeau JL. Treatment of obesity in polycystic ovary syndrome: a position statement of the Androgen Excess and Polycystic Ovary Syndrome Society 2008.

35. Keller J, Subramanyam L, Simha V, Gustofson R, Minjarez D, Garg A. Fertility and obstetrical complications in women with LMNA-related familial partial lipodystrophy. J Clin Endocrinol Metab 2009; 93:2223–2229.

36. Li Chen, Ling-Min Hu, YU-Feng Wang, Hai-Yan Yang, Xiao-Yang Huang: Genome-wide association study for SNPs associated with PCOS in human patients; 2017 Nov; 14(5): 4896–4900.

37. McAllister Jan M., Richard S. Legro, Bhavi P. Modi, Jerome F. Strauss: Functional Genomics of PCOS: From GWAS to Molecular Mechanisms 2015 Mar; 26(3):118–124.

38. Zawadski JK, Dunaif A. Diagnostic criteria for polycystic ovary syndrome; towards a rational approach. In: Dunaif A, Givens JR, Haseltine F, editors. Polycystic ovary syndrome. Vol. 1992. Boston, MA: Black-well Scientific; 1992. pp. 377–84.

Decoding the Genetics of PCOS

Abha Singh, Astha Srivastava

DEFINITION AND DIAGNOSTIC CRITERIA OF PCOS

Polycystic ovary syndrome (PCOS) is one of the most common human endocrine–metabolic disorders. The estimated prevalence is about 6–10% of reproductive age women and is characterized by hyperandrogenism and oligo- or amenorrhea.[1]

Symptoms of PCOS include hyperandrogenism, ovulatory dysfunction, polycystic ovarian morphology and gonadotropic abnormalities. In about two-thirds of affected individuals, PCOS is also associated with insulin resistance, compensatory hyperinsulinism and increased risk of metabolic morbidities, including diabetes mellitus, the metabolic syndrome, cerebrovascular disease and possibly cardiovascular disease.

Currently, the diagnosis of PCOS is based on the criteria of the ESRHE/ASRM Rotterdam consensus meeting held in 2003.[2] It based on at least two of the following features: Oligo- or anovulation, hyperandrogenism and polycystic ovaries by ultrasound. The Androgen Excess Society (AES) criteria require clinical and/or biochemical hyperandrogenism simultaneously with oligo-/anovulation and ultrasonographic evidence of polycystic ovaries.[3]

PCOS is a multifactorial disorder with interplay of various genetic, metabolic, endocrine and environmental abnormalities.[4] There is increasing evidence to suggest that PCOS affects the entire life of a woman, beginning right there *in utero* in genetically predisposed subjects, it manifests clinically at puberty, continues during the reproductive years. It can lead to wide range of adverse sequelae such as increased risk of cardiovascular disease, hypertension, diabetes and other metabolic complications like dyslipidemia. During the fertile period, it may cause anovulatory infertility and in pregnant it could be associated with increased prevalence of gestational complications, such as miscarriage, gestational diabetes and pre-eclampsia. Early diagnosis of PCOS is, therefore, essential to reduce the risk of such complications.

Diagnostic work-up includes hormonal evaluation of androgen levels, clinical evaluation of hirsutism through Ferriman-Gallwey score and ultrasonographic examination of the number of antral follicles and ovarian volume.

Genetics

The pathogenesis of PCOS is not clear, but familial clustering of cases suggests genetic involvement. Even within affected families, there is heterogeneity in presentation between sisters with polycystic ovaries. This variability of presentation of cases can be attributed to the interaction of a small number of genes with each other and with environmental (mainly nutritional) factors. The inherited basis of PCOS was established by twin studies as well as studies in first-degree relatives of women affected by PCOS clearly indicate genetic basis of this disorder.[5] A polygenic multifactorial model involving multiple genes is most likely the mode of inheritance.

The Dutch twin family study documented monozygotic correlation of 71% and a dizygotic correlation of 38%. In this study, it was estimated that genetic influences account for as much as 70% of the variance in the pathogenesis of PCOS.[5] 5- to 6-fold increase in the incidence of PCOS among first-degree female relatives of affected patients when compared with the prevalence of PCOS in general population has been shown in a study thus supporting genetic basis of PCOS (Kahsar-Miller et al).[6]

Only a few PCOS susceptibility genes have been validated despite advances in genetic technologies. Numerous candidate gene association studies have been conducted, but only a few genes have been consistently replicated in follow-up studies.[7]

The main candidate genes are those encoding for factors involved in regulating gonadotropin secretion and action, ovarian folliculogenesis, insulin secretion and action, weight and energy regulation, and androgen biosynthesis and action.

Despite the heterogeneity of PCOS, there are a number of well-characterized biochemical abnormalities which can provide a sound basis for adopting a candidate gene approach to the identification of susceptibility loci.

Various genome-wide association studies (GWAS) have been performed to identify putative gene targets. In the first genome-wide association and replication studies of PCOS conducted in Chinese Han individuals,[8] three loci were identified that were significantly associated with PCOS: two loci on chromosome 2 and a third locus on chromosome 9. One of these loci, on chromosome 2p16.3, contains the gene for the LH/hCG receptor (*LHCGR*), a logical susceptibility gene for PCOS. Two of the three 2p21 and 9p33.3, contained multiple single-nucleotide polymorphisms (SNPs) that appeared to be independently associated with PCOS. The chromosome 2p21 locus contained SNPs in *THADA*, a gene that codes for a thyroid

adenoma-associated protein. GWAS in Han Chinese individuals identified total of eleven PCOS candidate loci: *DENND1A, INSR, YAP1, C9orf3, RAB5B, HMGA2, TOX3, SUMO1P1/ ZNF217, THADA, FSHR and LHCGR*.[8, 9] Four studies in European populations published soon thereafter confirmed the association of several of these loci, including the FSHR/ LHCGR, DENND1A loci, as well as RAB5B and THADA.[10]

DENND1A locus at 9q22.32 has been recognized as a strong PCOS susceptibility gene as it has been replicated both in Asian and European populations.[10] DENND1A plays a key role in the hyperandrogenemia associated with PCOS.

Gonadotropin Secretion and Action

Altered LH action appears to be involved in the pathogenesis of PCOS, as illustrated by the following:

- PCOS patients often have higher serum LH concentrations and increased LH pulse frequency and amplitude. However, serum LH tends to be lower in obese women with PCOS compared with their lean counterparts.

- LH action at the ovarian level may be enhanced in PCOS as the LH receptor is overexpressed in thecal and granulosa cells from polycystic ovaries.

- Genetic variants of the LH beta-subunit and loci near *FSHR, LHCGR,* and *FSHB* in GWAS have been reported in patients with PCOS.

The *LHCGR* gene codes for a G-protein-coupled receptor for LH and human chorionic gonadotropin (hCG). In the ovary, induction of the *LHCGR* during granulosa cell differentiation is responsible for the pre-ovulatory follicle to respond to the mid-cycle LH surge resulting in ovulation. In women, inactivating mutations of *LHCGR* are associated with increased LH levels, enlarged ovaries and oligomenorrhea. *LHCGR* variants have been found to be associated with PCOS in some studies.[11, 12]

The increased LH to FSH ratio further enhances hypersecretion of androgens in the theca cells in the ovarian follicles. The increase in follicular androgens impairs follicular development and reduces the normal inhibition of gonadotropin-releasing hormone (GnRH) pulse frequency by progesterone, further promoting the development of the PCOS phenotype. Furthermore, increased LH pulses and enhanced daytime LH pulse secretion are observed early during puberty in girls with hyperandrogenism, suggesting that abnormalities in the pulsatile release of GnRH might underlie the development of PCOS, at least in some patients.

Dysfunction in Ovarian Folliculogenesis

In PCOS, the selection of a dominant follicle is abnormal, a consequence of insufficient FSH stimulation and local inhibition of FSH action, possibly due to excess local AMH and other intraovarian factors that modulate follicular recruitment and growth.

The Follistatin Gene

Urbanek et al.[13] examined the follistatin locus on chromosome 5, and found strong evidence for linkage with PCOS. However, further follow-up data from the same group did not find significant association when further families are added to the database.[14] However, there is a possibility that this and other genes implicated in folliculogenesis may have causal role in this disorder, which is, after all, characterized by disordered follicle development.

Furthermore, in PCOS, ovarian theca cells may be more sensitive to the effects of LH.

Insulin Secretion and Action

Overall, 50 to 70% of women with PCOS demonstrate clinically measurable insulin resistance *in vivo*, above and beyond that determined by their body weight (i.e. degree of obesity). Insulin stimulates theca cell secretion of androgens and inhibits hepatic sex hormone-binding globulin (SHBG) production, resulting in an increase in free androgens.

The Insulin Gene (INS) and Insulin Receptor (INSR)

The INSR plays a significant role in insulin metabolism and can play a critical role in PCOS pathogenesis via insulin resistance.[8]

Insulin gene (INS) variable number tandem repeat (VNTR) has been seen as a major susceptibility locus for PCOS.[15] The INS-VNTR lies in the 5-regulatory region of the gene; it has been shown to be involved in regulation of insulin gene expression and has been implicated in the etiology of type 2 diabetes. Franks et al.[16] found that class III alleles in the VNTR were associated with anovulatory PCOS in two independent populations and using two different methods of analysis (case-control studies and by use of affected family based controls; AFBAC).

They also established that there was excess allele sharing at the INS-VNTR locus. The geometric mean of fasting serum insulin concentrations was significantly higher in families in which linkage was demonstrated than without evidence of linkage.[15] This suggests a functional role for the VNTR variant in the expression of hyperinsulinemia/insulin resistance in PCOS. These data were extended by Ong et al.[17] In contrast, Urbanek et al.[13] found no evidence for excess allele sharing at this locus in their population.

The importance of insulin signaling in PCOS is also evident through the HAIR-AN syndrome (hyperandrogenism, insulin resistance, acanthosis nigricans), which is a subphenotype of PCOS characterized by severe insulin resistance.[18] Mutations in the insulin receptor gene, especially in the tyrosine kinase domain have been implicated in HAIR-AN syndrome.[19]

The etiology for the increased insulin resistance and, consequently, the hyperinsulinism in PCOS remains unclear. A post-binding defect in receptor signaling that selectively affects metabolic, but not mitogenic, pathways in classic insulin target tissues, such as adipose tissue and muscle (and possibly ovary), has been described.[20] These defects seem to affect glucose transporter 4 (GLUT4) expression. Additionally, epigenetic dysfunction may play a role in the insulin resistance of PCOS.

Weight and Energy Regulation

The presence of obesity worsens insulin resistance, the degree of hyperinsulinemia, the severity of ovulatory and menstrual dysfunction, and pregnancy outcome in PCOS. There is also proved association of obesity with an increased prevalence of metabolic syndrome, glucose intolerance, cardiovascular risk factors, and sleep apnea.

Androgen Biosynthesis and Action

Hyperandrogenism is a central feature for most forms (phenotypes) of PCOS. The androgens are secreted primarily by ovaries and secondarily by the adrenals.

The hyperandrogenemia is widely believed to be primarily of ovarian theca cell origin, although the adrenal zona reticularis contributes androgens, mainly dehydroepiandrosterone (DHEA), in approximately 25% of cases. Although hyperinsulinism is associated with hyperandrogenism in PCOS, insulin resistance alone is not sufficient for the development of PCOS, suggesting that an underlying (genetic) predisposition to hyperandrogenism must also be present. Genes implicated in the pathway of androgen production and metabolism include those encoding the major endocrine regulator, LH, its receptor, key P450 steroidogenic enzymes such as cholesterol side chain cleavage (P450scc), 17 α-hydroxylase/17, 20-lyase (P450c17α). Also considered is CYP19, encoding P450 aromatase which is responsible for the conversion of androgen to estrogen in granulosa cells.

CYP11a

Adrenal and ovarian steroidogeneses start with the conversion of cholesterol to progesterone, which is catalyzed by P450 cytochrome side chain cleavage enzyme encoded by CYP11a located at 15q24. This conversion is the rate limiting step of steroidogenesis. Earlier studies had proposed that allelic variants of CYP11a have a role in the etiology of hyperandrogenemia and/or PCOS, subsequent studies have failed to find a significant linkage or association between this gene locus and/or its alleles and PCOS.[21–23] A polymorphic sequence, a pentanucleotide repeat *(tttta)n*, at position–528 from the ATG initiation codon in the 52-region of the CYP11a gene, seems to be associated with PCOS susceptibility. Further research is needed to confirm these controversial results.

CYP21

Conversion of 17-hydroxyprogesterone into 11-deoxycortisol is catalyzed by the 21-hydroxylase enzyme encoded by CYP21. The deficiency of this enzyme, which is inherited as an autosomal recessive trait, is responsible for most cases of congenital adrenal hyperplasia although CYP21 and its associated mutations have no role to play in the development of PCOS.

CYP17

Conversion of pregnenolone and progesterone into 17-hydroxypregnenolone and 17-hydroxyprogesterone, respectively, and of these steroids into dehydroepiandrosterone and androstenedione, is catalyzed by the P450c17α enzyme. This enzyme has both 17α-hydroxylase and 17,20-lyase activities and is encoded by CYP17 located at 10q24.3. It has been proclaimed that the P450c17 enzyme activity and expression increases in ovary theca cells of women with PCOS.[13]

CYP19

CYP19 converts androgen to estrogen. The enzyme complex is composed of cytochrome P450 aromatase and NADPH cytochrome

P450 reductase, and P450 aromatase is encoded by CYP19 located at 15p21.1. Aromatase activity might be decreased in PCOS follicles and the excess androgen leads to the improper follicle development.[24]

Hydroxysteroid Dehydrogenase

HSD17B1 and HSD17B2 belong to the group of alcohol oxidoreductase, which catalyze the dehydrogenation of 17-hydroxysteroids during steroidogenesis. A higher level of expression of mRNA synthesizing and inactivating enzyme has been reported in women with PCOS. HSD3B deficiency in hyperandrogenic females (HF) has been to insulinresistant polycystic ovary syndrome.[25]

DENND1A and its Association with PCOS

DENND1A has gained recognition as a strong PCOS susceptibility gene. The association of the DENND1A locus in PCOS has been confirmed in populations of European ancestry in multiple studies.[26]

GWAS studies have consistently identified SNPs near the gene *DENND1A* as potential PCOS loci. In a study of theca cells of normal and PCOS women, the DENND1A protein was found to be located in the cytoplasm as well as nuclei of theca cells, suggesting a possible role in gene regulation. DENND1A immune staining was more intense in the theca of PCOS ovaries. The DENND1A variant 2 (DENND1A.V2) protein and mRNA levels were found to be increased in PCOS theca cells, and exosomal DENND1A.V2 RNA was significantly elevated in urine from PCOS women compared with normal-cycling women. The expression of DENND1A in well-characterized theca cells from normal cycling and PCOS women was studied by Jan M. McAllister.[26] In their study, they found that forced expression of DENND1A.V2 in normal theca cells increases CYP17A1 and CYP11A1 gene expression and converts the cells to a PCOS phenotype of augmented androgen and progestin biosynthesis.

In contrast, knock-down of DENND1A.V2 with silencing shRNA plasmids or lentivirus in PCOS theca cells reverts the cells to a normal phenotype of reduced CYP17A1 and CYP11A1 gene expression and androgen and progestin biosynthesis. From these observations, they concluded that DENND1A is involved in a signaling cascade that augments transcription of steroidogenic genes that subsequently results in increased androgen production.

Their observation was that augmented CYP17 and CYP11A mRNA and androgen biosynthesis in PCOS theca cells can be reduced using DENND1A.V2-specific IgG. They concluded that this observation raises the possibility that humanized monoclonal antibodies against DENND1A.V2 may be a useful biologic therapeutic agents for the hyperandrogenemia associated with PCOS, and possibly other phenotypes related to insulin action.

Environmental Factors

The most clearly defined environmental factor likely affecting the development of PCOS is diet and its association with obesity.

REFERENCES

1. Goodarzi MO, Dumesic DA, Chazenbalk G, Azziz R. Polycystic ovary syndrome: etiology, pathogenesis and diagnosis. Nat Rev Endocrinol. 2011; 7(4):219–31. doi: 10.1038/nrendo.2010.217 PMID: 21263450.

2. The Rotterdam ESHRE/ASRM-sponsored PCOS consensus workshop group. Revised 2003 consensus on diagnostic criteria and long-term health risks related to polycystic ovary syndrome (PCOS). Hum Reprod 2004; 19:41–47.

3. Azziz R, Carmina E, Dewailly D, et al. Criteria for defining polycystic ovary syndrome as a predominantly hyperandrogenic syndrome: An Androgen Excess guideline. J Clin Endocrinol Metab 2006; 91:4237–45.

4. Franks S, Mc Carthy M, Hardy K. Development of polycystic ovary syndrome: involvement of genetic and environmental factors. Int J Androl 2006; 29:278–85.

5. Vink JM, Sadrzadeh S, Lambalk CB, Boomsma DI. Heritability of polycystic ovary syndrome in a Dutch twin-family study. J Clin Endocrinol Metab 2006; 91:2100.

6. Kahsar-Miller MD, Nixon C, Boots LR, et al. Prevalence of polycystic ovary syndrome (PCOS) in first-degree relatives of patients with PCOS. Fertil Steril 2001; 75:53.

7. Strauss JF 3rd, et al. Persistence pays off for PCOS gene prospectors. The Journal of Clinical Endocrinology and Metabolism 2012; 97:2286–88. [PubMed: 22774210]

8. Chen ZJ, et al. Genome-wide association study identifies susceptibility loci for polycystic ovary syndrome on chromosome 2p16.3–2p21 and 9q33.3. Nat Genet 2011; 43:55–59. [PubMed: 21151128]

9. Shi Y, et al. Genome-wide association study identifies eight new risk loci for polycystic ovary syndrome. Nat Genet 2012; 44:1020–25. [PubMed: 22885925]

10. Goodarzi MO, et al. Replication of association of DENND1A and THADA variants with poly-cystic ovary syndrome in European cohorts. J Med Genet 2012; 49:90–95. [PubMed: 22180642]

11. Mutharasan P, et al. Evidence for chromosome 2p16.3 polycystic ovary syndrome susceptibility locus in affected women of European ancestry. The Journal of Clinical Endocrinology and Metabolism 2013; 98:E185–E190. [PubMed: 23118426]

12. Liu N, et al. Association of the genetic variants of luteinizing hormone, luteinizing hormone receptor and polycystic ovary syndrome. Reproductive Biology and Endocrinology: RB and E 2012; 10:36.

13. Urbanek M, Legro RS, DriscollDA, Azziz R, Ehrmann DA, Norman RJ, Strauss JF, Spielman RS, Dunaif A. Thirty-seven candidate genes for polycystic ovary syndrome: Strongest evidence for linkage is with follistatin. Proc Natl Acad Sci USA 1999; 96:8573–78.

14. Urbanek M, Proceedings of "Polycystic Ovary Syndrome: Basic Biology and Clinical Interven-tion," National Institute of Environmental of Health Sciences (NIH), Sept. 2000.

15. Waterworth DM, Bennett ST, Gharani N, McCarthy MI, Hague S, Batty S, Conway GS, White D, Todd JA, Franks S, Williamson R. Linkage and association of insulin gene VNTR regulatory polymorphism with polycystic ovary syndrome. Lancet 1997; 349:986–990.

16. Stephen Franks, Mark McCarthy. Reviews in Endocrine and Metabolic Disorders 2004; 5:69–76.

17. Ong KK, Phillips DI, Fall C, Poulton J, Bennett ST, Golding J, Todd JA, Dunger DB. The insulin gene VNTR, type 2 diabetes and birth weight. Nat Genet 1999; 21:262–263.

18. Rager KM, Omar HA. Androgen excess dis-orders in women: the severe insulin-resistant hyperandrogenic syndrome, HAIR-AN. The Scientific World Journal. 2006; 6:116–21.

19. Globerman H, Karnieli E. Analysis of the insulin receptor gene tyrosine kinase domain in obese patients with hyperandrogenism, insulin resistance and acanthosis nigricans (type C insulin resistance). International Journal of Obesity and Related Metabolic Disorders 1998; 22:349–53. [PubMed: 9578241]

20. Diamanti-Kandarakis E, Dunaif A. Insulin resistance and the polycystic ovary syndrome revisited: an update on mechanisms and implications. Endocr Rev 2012; 33:981.

21. Gharani N, Waterworth DM, Batty S, et al. Association of the steroid synthesis gene CYP11a with polycystic ovary syndrome and hyper-androgenism. Hum Mol Genet 1997; 6:397–402.

22. Diamanti-Kandarakis E, Bartzis MI, Bergiele AT, et al. Microsatellite polymorphism (tttta)(n) at – 528 base pairs of gene CYP11alpha influences hyperandrogenemia in patients with polycystic ovary syndrome. Fertil Steril 2000; 73:735–41.

23. Gaasenbeek M, Powell BL, Sovio U, et al. Large-scale analysis of the relationship between CYP11A promoter variation, polycystic ovarian syndrome, and serum testosterone. J Clinl Endocrino Metab 2004; 89:2408–13.

24. Prapas N, Karkanaki A, Prapas I, Kalogiannidis I, Katsikis I, Panidis D. Genetics ofpolycystic ovary syndrome. Hippokratia 2009; 13(4):216–23.

25. Blomquist CH. Kinetic analysis of enzymic activities: prediction of multiple forms of 17 beta-hydroxysteroid dehydrogenase. J Steroid Biochem Mol Biol 1995; 55:515–24.

26. McAllister JM et al. Over expression of a DENND1A isoform produces a polycystic ovary syndrome theca phenotype. Proc Natl Acad Sci USA 2004; 111:E1519–E1527.

PCOS and Autoimmunity

Kiran Pandey, Pavika Lal

INTRODUCTION

Polycystic ovarian syndrome (PCOS) is a reproductive-endocrine-metabolic disorder that affects the entire lifespan of a woman-from womb to tomb and has become a public health issue of great concern (Fig. 1.1). PCOS was first described by Stein and Leventhal in 1935 (also known as Stein-Leventhal syndrome) and results from a functional derangement that develops when a chronic anovulatory state persists for a sufficient length of time. This heterogenous complex multifaceted disorder may significantly impact the quality of life of a woman during her reproductive years, and also contributing to morbidity and mortality by the time of menopause by predisposing to increased risk of CVD, type II diabetes mellitus and endometrial cancer.

PREVALENCE

This enigmatic disorder is galloping into epidemic proportions and its incidence is clearly on the rise, globally. It is the most common endocrinopathy among females of reproductive age group. Worldwide prevalence estimates of PCOS are highly variable, ranging from 2.2% to as high as 26%.[1] In India, experts claim 10% of the women to be affected by PCOS and yet no proper published statistical data on the prevalence of PCOS in India is available.[2] Urban middle class women are more predisposed to PCOS due to constant health pressures of globalization, economic liberalizations, sedentary lifestyle and access to high calorie food and machineries for all household work leading to higher prevalence of PCOS as compared to rural women who still lead a traditional lifestyle.[2]

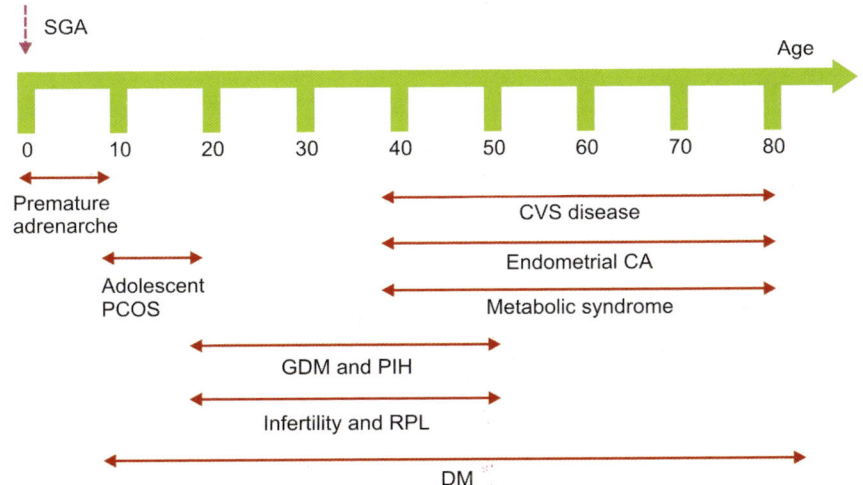

Fig. 3.1: Consequences of PCOS spectrum is seen across entire lifespan of a woman

Incidence of PCOS varies not only by the definition used (approximately 1 in 12 women of reproductive age), but also differs as per the presenting symptoms, e.g. menstrual cycle disturbance (70%), obesity (50%), hirsutism (70%), androgenic alopecia (10%) and acne (30%).[3]

may present with a single overt clinical symptom like menstrual disorder or social embarrassing manifestations like acne or hirsutism (Fig. 3.3.) However, this may be only the tip of the iceberg where the other subclinical (pre-disease) conditions may be a larger part of the submerged portion of the iceberg.

CLINICAL PRESENTATION

PCOS is a challenging disease both for the gynecologist as well as endocrinologist with its diverse clinical presentations with differing severity (Fig. 3.2). A given PCOS individual

DIAGNOSTIC CRITERIA OF PCOS[4–6]

PCOS is currently known to be a genetically complex endocrine disorder of uncertain etiology with a complicated pathophysiology (Figs 3.4 to 3.6).

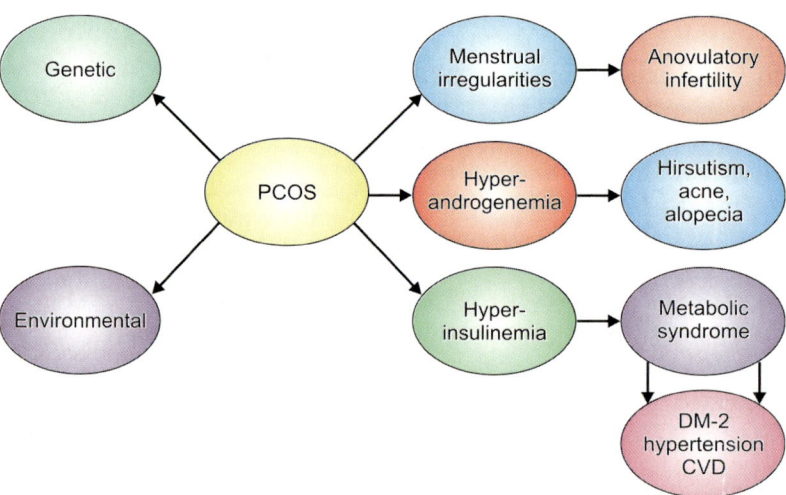

Fig. 3.2: Clinical features of PCOS

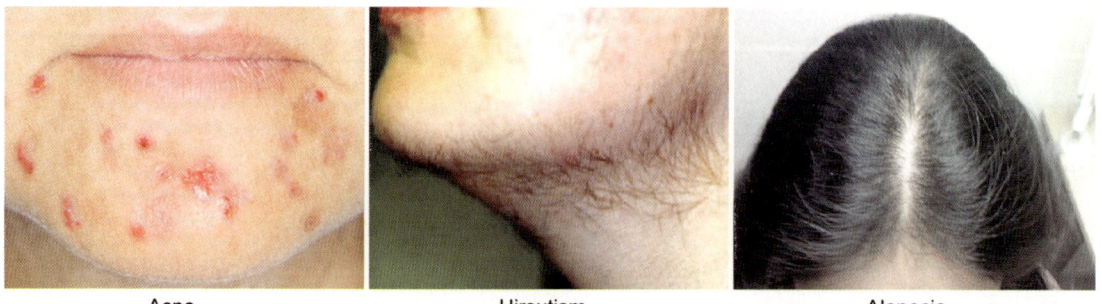

Acne   Hirsutism   Alopecia

Fig. 3.3: Physical signs of PCOS

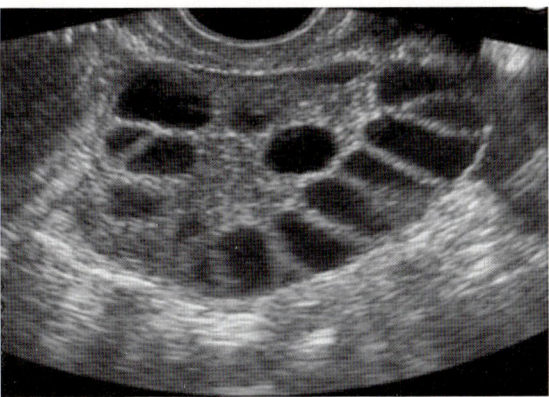

Fig. 3.4: USG showing pearl necklace appearance of PCOS

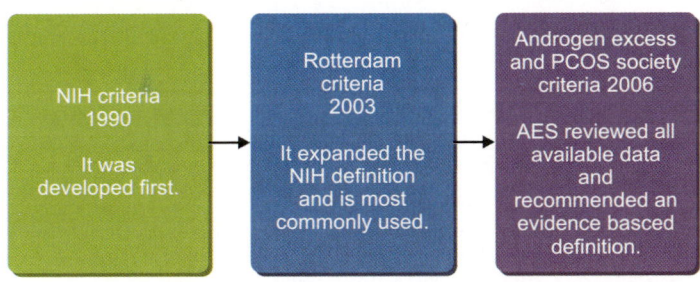

Fig. 3.5: Different criteria for PCOS

None of the criteria addressed insulin resistance and metabolic manifestations.

PCOS definition NIH criteria 1990	Rotterdam criteria 2003 (ESHRE/ASHRM)	AES criteria (2006)
Patient demonstrates both: 1. Clinical and/or biochemical signs of hyperandrogenism 2. Oligo- or chronic anovulation	Two of the following three manifestations: 1. Irregular or absent ovulation 2. Hyperandrogenism (clinical or biochemical) 3. Polycystic ovarian morphology on USG	Patient demonstrates both: 1. Hirsutism and/or hyperandrogenemia (clinical or biochemical) 2. Oligo-/anovulation and/or polycystic ovarian morphology *Azziz et al. JCEM 2006; 91:4237–45*
Exclude other etiologies of androgen excess		

Fig. 3.6: Different criteria for PCOS

Other etiologies of androgen excess include:
- Adult onset adrenal hyperplasia (AOAH)
- Cushing's syndrome
- Androgen producing tumor—ovary or adrenal
- Hyper- or hypogonadotropic disorders
- Hyperprolactinemia
- Thyroid disorders

Why the need to describe Phenotypes?

PCOS has always remained a debatable topic among clinician and scientists worldwide. The

NIH criteria were criticized for reflecting majority opinion rather than clinical trial data[7] and for their omission of ultrasonographic evidence of polycystic ovaries (PCO) that many considered a definitive marker of PCOS. The **'Rotterdam criteria'** was intended to reflect the clinical heterogeneity of PCOS but were criticized for being too expensive.[6, 7]

The AE-PCOS Society and Rotterdam described various phenotypes of PCOS which is important for stratification of risk evaluation and treatment accordingly (Fig. 3.7).

Characteristics of different phenotypes: The spectrum of clinical and biochemical features found in various phenotypes of PCOS are depicted in Table 3.1.[7–11]

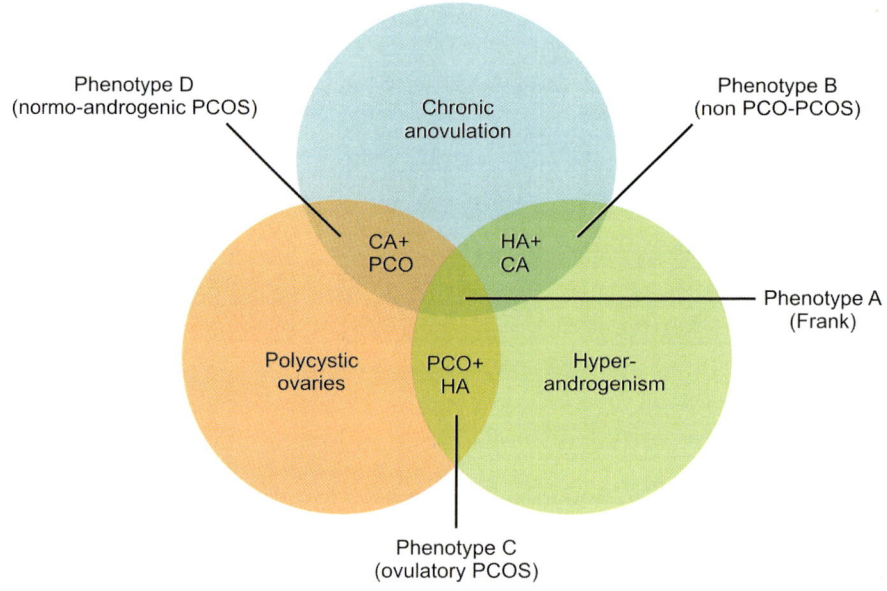

Fig. 3.7: Clinical phenotypes of PCOS

TABLE 3.1: Clinical and biochemical features of PCOS

	Androgens	LH/FSH	Insulin resistance	CV risk	PCOM	Menstrual problems
Type 1/classic PCOS/phenotype A	Increased	Increased	Increased	Increased	+	Oligo
Type 2/non-PCO PCOS/phenotype B	Increased	Mild increase	Increased	Increased	−	Oligo
Ovulatory PCOS/ phenotype C	Increased	Normal	Mild increase	Mild increase	+	Regular
Normo-androgenic PCOS/phenotype D	Normal	Increased	Normal	Normal	+	Oligo

PCOM: Polycystic ovarian morphology

PATHOPHYSIOLOGY OF PCOS

A comprehensive and detailed explanation of PCOS is lacking and its complexity involves multiple pathophysiological mechanisms but the definition of each contributing factor has been slow to emerge. **PCOS occurs as a result of a 'vicious cycle', which can be initiated at any one of many entry points leading to ovarian androgen excess and anovulation.**

Several theories have been proposed to explain the pathogenesis of PCOS:[11]

1. A unique defect in insulin action and secretion that leads to hyperinsulinemia and insulin resistance by several mechanisms (Fig. 3.8):
   - Peripheral target tissue resistance
   - Decreased hepatic clearance
   - Increased pancreatic sensitivity.

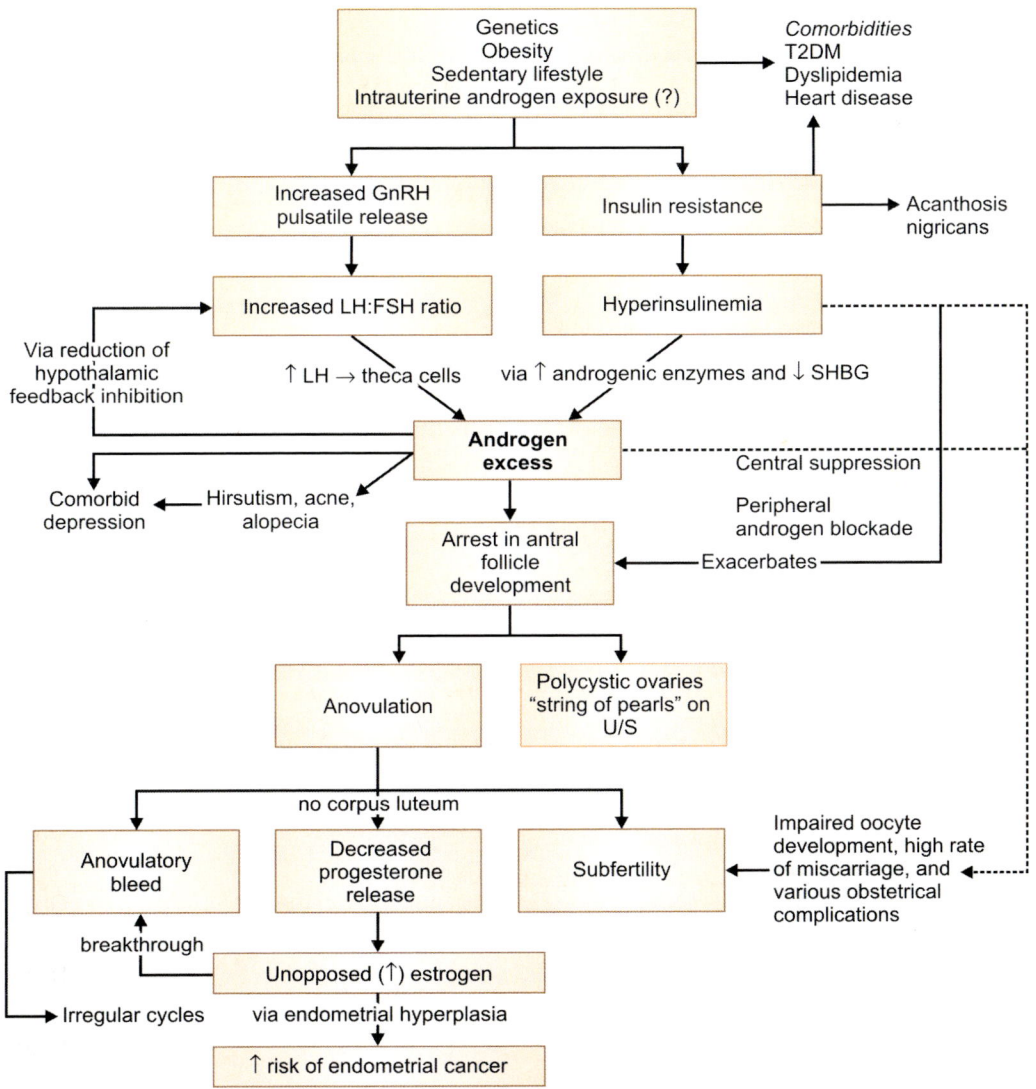

Fig. 3.8: Mechanisms leading to PCOS[12]

2. Hyperinsulinemia also augments androgen production in PCOS resulting in **hyperandrogenemia**. Insulin acts by:

   - Directly, as a cogonadotropin augmenting LH activity through stimulation of ovarian receptors of insulin and insulin-like growth factors.

   - Indirectly, by enhancing the amplitude of serum LH pulses.

3. A **primary neuroendocrine defect leading to an exaggerated LH pulse frequency and amplitude** (LH hypersecretion) both basally and in response to GnRH administration, is a characteristic hallmark of PCOS. Elevated LH levels due to:

   - Increased sensitivity of the pituitary to GnRH stimulation

   - Reduction in hypothalamic opioid inhibition because of the chronic absence of progesterone.

     – **In PCOS, LH/GnRH pulses are persistently rapid and favor LH synthesis, hyperandrogenemia and impaired follicular maturation.**

4. A defect of androgen synthesis that results in enhanced ovarian theca cells androgen production.

5. An increased peripheral cortisol metabolism resulting in enhanced adrenal androgen production.

LOW GRADE CHRONIC INFLAMMATION IN PCOS

Low grade chronic inflammation has been proposed recently as a novel mechanism in the pathogenesis of PCOS substantiated by increased CRP concentration as well as other inflammatory markers in such patients compared to normal female (Fig. 3.9).

C Reactive Protein

- C reactive protein is one of the most important marker as well as mediator of inflammatory processes. It is an **acute phase reactant produced by hepatocytes** under the stimulatory control of proinflammatory cytokines such as interleukin-6 (IL-6) and tumor necrosis factor-α (TNF-α).[13, 14]

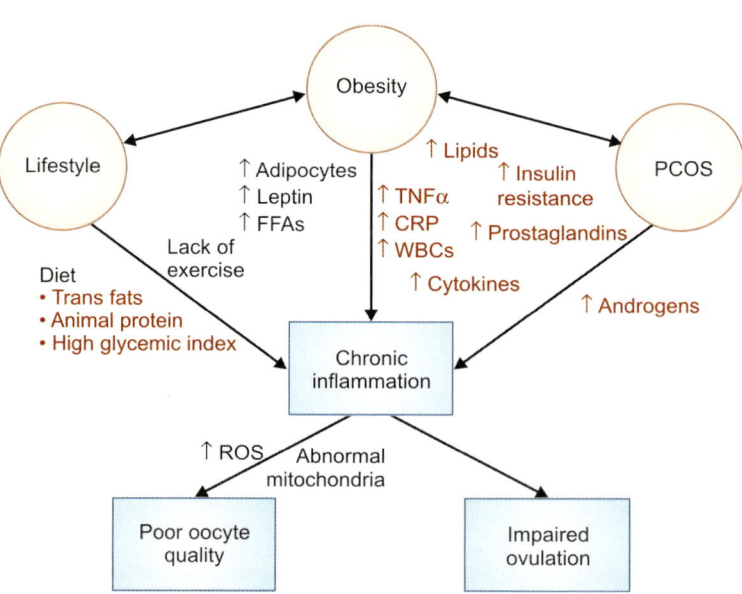

Fig. 3.9: The vicious cycle of PCOS and chronic inflammation

- Recent meta-analysis evaluated 31 clinical trials and included 2,359 women with PCOS and 1,289 controls.[15] It concluded that **CRP in women with PCOS is on average 96%** (95% CI: 71–122%) greater than in healthy subjects.

Proinflammatory Cytokines and Chemokines

- Chronic inflammatory processes are associated with elevations of a host of proinflammatory cytokines and chemokines including **IL-18, monocyte chemoattractant protein-1 (MCP-1) and macrophage inflammatory protein-1α (MIP-1α)** and their elevation are seen in PCOS individuals.[16–18]
- Action of chemokines:
  - MCP-1 plays a major role in the development of atherosclerosis[19]
  - MIP-1α for recruitment and activation of leukocytes[20]
  - IL-18 is closely related to insulin resistance and metabolic syndrome and serum level of IL-18 correlates with total testosterone level and inversely with insulin sensitivity index.[21]

White Blood Cells (WBCs)

WBC in women with PCOS correlated with insulin resistance determined by the homeostasis model (HOMA). Elevation of WBC in women with PCOS was subsequently confirmed in various studies.[21, 22]

Oxidative Stress

Oxidative stress and chronic inflammation are closely inter-related; indeed, extensive evidence supports the concept of a vicious cycle, whereby inflammation induces generation of reactive oxygen species (ROS), while oxidative stress promotes and aggravates inflammation.[23]

Advanced Glycation End-products

Advanced glycation end-products (AGEs) are generated by non-enzymatic reactions between reducing sugars and amino groups of proteins forming reversible Schiff bases, Amadori products and, ultimately, reactive cross-linked derivative molecules. AGEs act on signal-transducing receptors **(RAGE)** leading to induction of oxidative stress. AGEs, by acting both directly and through RAGE promote development and progression of cardiovascular disease.[24]

Chronic low grade inflammation has emerged as a key contributor to the pathogenesis of PCOS which increased risk for insulin resistance, cardiovascular disease as well as infertility in such patients.[25]

LEAKY GUT SYNDROME AND PCOS

What is Leaky Gut Syndrome?

The intestinal epithelial lining along with basement membrane and mucin secreted by goblet cells, forms a protective barrier that separates the host from the antigenic sources (high fat and sugar diet) of environment. In pathologic conditions, the permeability of the epithelial lining may be compromised allowing the passage of toxins, antigens, and bacteria in the lumen to enter the bloodstream creating a 'leaky gut'. In individuals with a genetic predisposition, a leaky gut may allow environmental factors to enter the body and trigger the initiation and development of autoimmune diseases (Fig. 3.10).

Clinical conditions that have already been linked with dysbiosis of the gut microbiota and a 'leaky gut' are irritable bowel syndrome (IBS), inflammatory bowel disease (Crohn's disease, ulcerative colitis), and chronic fatigue syndrome (CFS) (Fig. 3.11).[26, 27]

Dysbiosis of gut microbiota, can result in the activation of the host's immune system, triggering a chronic inflammatory response that impairs insulin receptor function and initiates a state of insulin resistance. The resulting hyperinsulinemia interferes with follicular development, while driving excess androgen production by the theca cells of

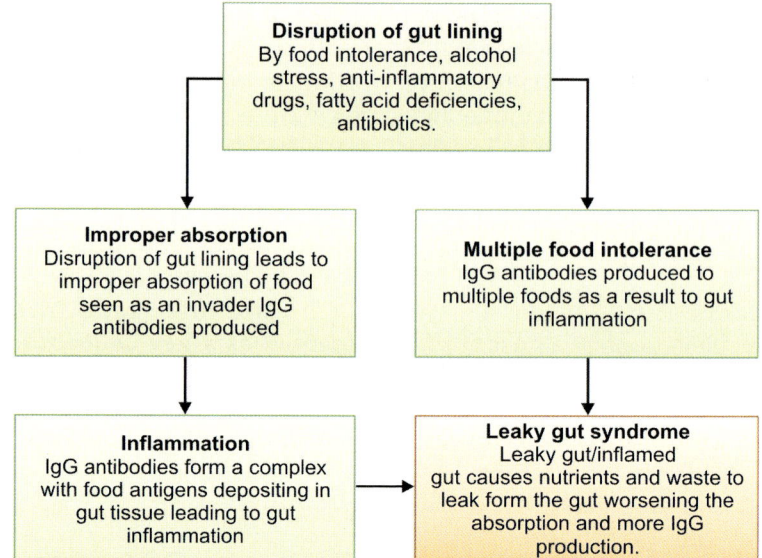

Disruption of gut lining
By food intolerance, alcohol stress, anti-inflammatory drugs, fatty acid deficiencies, antibiotics.

Improper absorption
Disruption of gut lining leads to improper absorption of food seen as an invader IgG antibodies produced

Multiple food intolerance
IgG antibodies produced to multiple foods as a result to gut inflammation

Inflammation
IgG antibodies form a complex with food antigens depositing in gut tissue leading to gut inflammation

Leaky gut syndrome
Leaky gut/inflamed gut causes nutrients and waste to leak form the gut worsening the absorption and more IgG production.

Fig. 3.10: Weakening of various mechanical and biochemical barriers of the gut resulting in the passage of antigenic material into the bloodstream

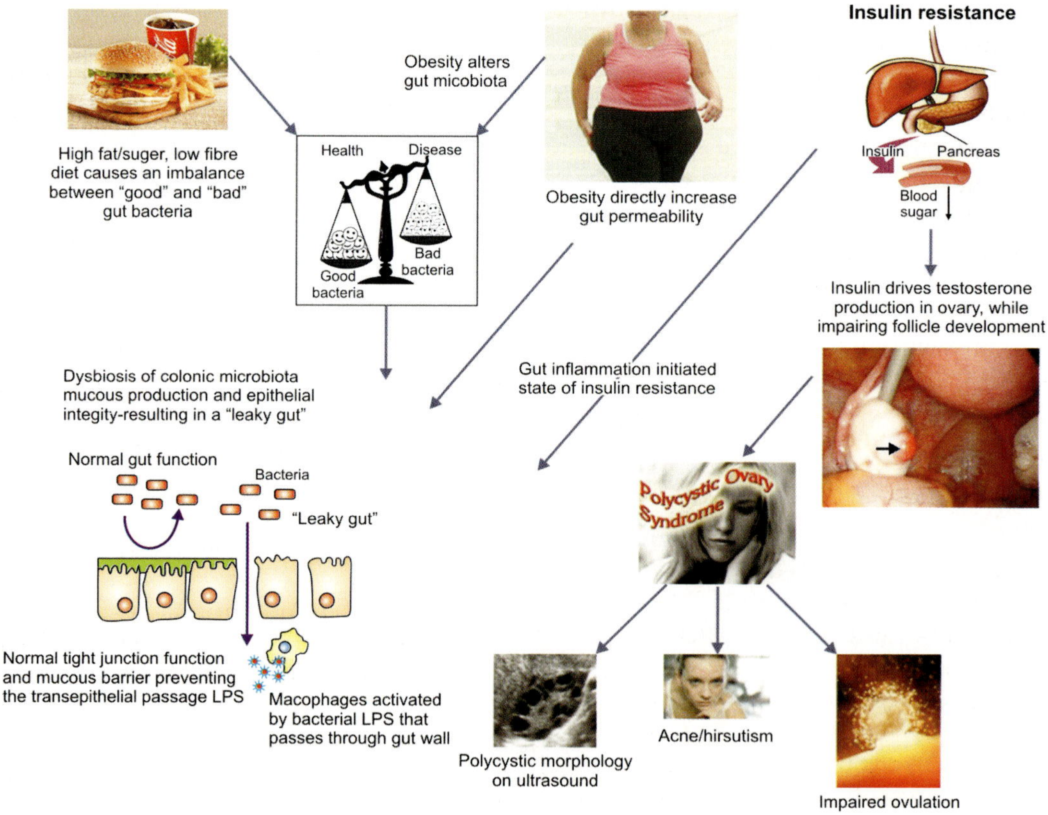

Insulin resistance

High fat/suger, low fibre diet causes an imbalance between "good" and "bad" gut bacteria

Obesity alters gut micobiota

Health   Disease

Good bacteria   Bad bacteria

Obesity directly increase gut permeability

Insulin   Pancreas

Blood sugar

Insulin drives testosterone production in ovary, while impairing follicle development

Dysbiosis of colonic microbiota mucous production and epithelial integity-resulting in a "leaky gut"

Gut inflammation initiated state of insulin resistance

Normal gut function

Bacteria

"Leaky gut"

Polycystic Ovary Syndrome

Normal tight junction function and mucous barrier preventing the transepithelial passage LPS

Macophages activated by bacterial LPS that passes through gut wall

Polycystic morphology on ultrasound

Acne/hirsutism

Impaired ovulation

Fig. 3.11: Pathophysiology of leaky gut syndrome and PCOS[28]

ovary—thereby producing all three classical features of the PCOS. This novel microbiological paradigm for PCOS has been labeled as the **DOGMA theory.**

Evidence for Microbiological Dysbiosis and a 'Leaky Gut' in PCOS

The key pathophysiological links in the DOGMA theory of PCOS are twofold (Fig. 3.11).[29–35]

- **Firstly,** a diet high in saturated fat and refined sugars, commonly observed in overweight PCOS patients, is known to favor the growth of **'bad' gram-negative bacteria within the gut; while reducing the growth of beneficial 'good' bacteria such as** *Bifidobacteria* **and** *Lactobacillus.* The cell wall of gram-negative bacteria contains a powerful immunostimulant called lipopolysaccharide (LPS), which can cause profound activation of the innate immune system, if it is allowed to traverse the gut wall and enter the systemic circulation.

- **Secondly,** the high saturated fat-sugar/low fiber diet, as well as obesity per se, causes an increase in gut mucosal permeability, facilitating the transfer of LPS from the gut lumen into the circulation, initiating a state of 'metabolic endotoxemia'. The **resultant chronic activation of hepatic and tissue macrophages produces impaired insulin receptor function** and resulting insulin resistance.

PCOS AND AUTOIMMUNE RELATION

There is an association between PCOS and other autoimmune diseases like Graves' disease, Hashimoto's thyroiditis, type II diabetes mellitus and systemic lupus erythematosus. It has been implicated that low level of progesterone in PCOS causes overstimulation of immune system to produce more estrogen which leads to formation various antibodies.[36]

Autoantibodies in PCOS

1. Anti-nuclear Antibody (ANA)[37]

- Production of ANA—hallmark of autoimmune disorders due to exposure of antigens in:
  - Inflammation
  - Immune hyperstimulation
  - Process of tissue destruction
- Detection of ANA in autoimmune disorders like:
  - SLE (systemic lupus erythematosus)
  - Sjögren's syndrome
  - Polymyositis
  - Dermatomyositis
  - Autoimmune hepatitis.

2. Antithyroid Antibody[38, 39]

- Autoimmune thyroiditis produces autoantibodies against one or more components of thyroid.
- Antithyroid antibodies:
  - Antithyroid peroxidase (anti-TPO)
  - Thyrotrophic receptor (TRAbs)
  - Thyroglobulin antibodies

  } Associated with Hashimoto thyroiditis

Patrikova et al. has suggested strong association of antithyroid antibodies with PCOS, e.g. anti-TPO 7.81%.[40] **Kachuei et al.** reported strong association of anti-thyroglobulin (p = 0.275) and anti-TPO antibodies (p = 0.040) in PCOS patients.[41] **Arduc et al.** suggested association of anti-thyroglobulin (p = 0.039) and anti-TPO antibodies (p = 0.002) in PCOS.[42]

Janssen et al. suggested that autoimmune thyroiditis (AIT) is three times more common in PCOS as compared to non-PCOS women of reproductive age.[43] Sarkar reported strong association of infertility, miscarriages, and disturbed thyroid profile in pregnant females. Both hypo- and hyperthyroidism can lead to increased rate of miscarriages, fetal death, and late cognitive development of offsprings.[44]

3. Anti-Islet Cell Antibody[45]

Production of islet cell autoantibodies is due to the damaged pancreatic beta cell which cause hyperglycemia leading to increase in weight gain and ovarian hyperandrogenism.

These autoantibodies can be used to estimate an individual's risk of developing type I diabetes. **Gardener et al. reported anti-islet cell antibodies in 83% of PCOS patients.**[46]

CONCLUSION AND AVENUES FOR FUTURE RESEARCH

PCOS has been muddled up with lots of various etiological factors known for its complex behavior and notoriously influencing various organ systems out of which some are still hiding behind the shadow. Because of many experiments and studies, recently, autoimmunity has come to a spotlight for linking PCOS with numerous autoimmune factors. **They have shown the linkage of auto-antibodies in PCOS like ANA and anti-TPO which has unfolded a new field of research on molecular level.** The low grade chronic inflammatory mediators like CRP, WBCs, and MCP-1 have marked a new territory of association with PCOS. The DOGMA theory also accounts for gut microbiota in the pathogenesis of PCOS and, therefore, modulation of gut microbiota may prove beneficial for PCOS treatment. Considering the literature, **emphasis** should be given to the **role of auto-immunity, leaky gut syndrome, and low grade chronic inflammation and their relationships with obesity, hyperandrogenism and insulin resistance.** This will help us further improve and enhance the knowledge of clinicians about undiscovered diagnostic, preventive and curative interventions of women with PCOS.

REFERENCES

1. Kabel AM . Polycystic ovarian syndrome: insights into pathogenesis, diagnosis, prognosis, pharmacological and non-pharmacological treatment. Pharmacol. Rep 2016; 1(103) pp. E1-E5.

2. Vidya Bharathi R, Swetha S , NeerajaaJ , Varsha J Madhavica, Dakshina Moorthy Janani, SN Rekha, S Ramya, B Usha. An epidemiological survey: Effect of predisposing factors for PCOS in Indian urban and rural population. Middle East Fertility Society Journal 22 (2017) 313–316.

3. Roger Hart MD, FRANZCOG, MRCOG (Senior Lecturer in Obstetrics and Gynaecology) Martha Hickey MD, FRANZCOG, MRCOG (Associate Professor of Obstetrics and Gynaecology) Stephen Franks MD, FRCP, Hon MD, FRCOG (ad eundem), F Med Sci (Professor of Reproductive Endocrinology). Definitions, prevalence and symptoms of polycystic ovaries and polycystic ovary syndrome. Best Practice and Research Clinical Obstetrics and Gynaecology; Volume 18, Issue 5, October 2004, Pages 671–683.

4. Zawadzki JK, Dunaif A. Diagnostic Criteria for Polycystic Ovary Syndrome: Towards a Rational Approach, Polycystic Ovary Syndrome; Blackwell Scientific, Boston (1992), pp. 377–384.

5. Fr DD, Tarlatzis R. Recised 2003 consensus on diagnostic criteria and long-term health risks related to Polycystic ovary syndrome.

6. Azziz R, Carmina E, Dewailly D, et al. Criteria for defining polycystic ovary syndrome as a predominantly hyperandrogenic syndrome: an androgen excess society guideline. J.Clin. Endocrinol. Metab 2006; 91(11) pp. 4237–4245.

7. Azziz R. Diagnosis of polycystic ovarian syndrome: the Rotterdam criteria are premature. J Clin Endocrinol Metab 2006; 91(3):781–85.

8. Lujan M, Chizen D, Pierson R. Diagnostic criteria for polycystic ovary syndrome: pitfalls and controversies. J Obstet Gynecol Canada 2008; 30(8):671–79.

9. Norman RJ, Dewailly D, Legro RS, Hickey TE. Polycystic ovary syndrome. Lancet. 2007; 370(9588):685–697.

10. Moghetti P, Tosi F, Bonin C, et al. Divergences in insulin resistance between the different phenotypes of the polycystic ovary syndrome. J Clin Endocrinol Metab 2013; 98(4):E628-37.

11. Clinical Endocrinology (2004) 60, 1–17 doi: 10.1046/j.1365-2265.2003.01842.x © 2003 Blackwell Publishing Ltd 1 Blackwell Publishing Ltd. Review The pathophysiology of polycystic ovary syndrome Tasoula Tsilchorozidou, Caroline Overton and Gerard S. Conway Department of Endocrinology, University College London Hospitals, London, UK.

12. J Obstet Gynaecol Can. Polycystic Ovarian Syndrome (PCOS) 2010 May; 32(5):423–8.

13. Castell JV, Gomez-Lechon MJ, David M, Andus T, Geiger T, Trullenque R, et al. Interleukin-6 is the major regulator of acute phase protein synthesis in adult human hepatocytes. FEBS Lett 1989; 242:237–39.

14. Han KH, Hong KH, Park JH, Ko J, Kang DH, Choi KJ, et al. C-reactive protein promotes monocyte chemoattractant protein-1-mediated chemotaxis through upregulating CC chemokine receptor 2 expression in human monocytes. Circulation 2004; 109:2566–71.

15. Escobar-Morreale HF, Luque-Ramirez M, Gonzalez F. Circulating inflammatory markers in polycystic ovary syndrome: a systematic review and metaanalysis. Fertil Steril 2011; 95:1048–58.e1–2.

16. Yang Y, Qiao J, Li R, Li MZ. Is interleukin-18 associated with polycystic ovary syndrome? Reprod Biol Endocrinol 2011;9:7.

17. Gonzalez F, Rote NS, Minium J, Kirwan JP. Evidence of proatherogenic inflammation in polycystic ovary syndrome. Metabolism 2009; 58:954–62.

18. Glintborg D, Andersen M, Richelsen B, Bruun JM. Plasma monocyte chemoattractant protein-1 (MCP-1) and macrophage inflammatory protein-1 alpha are increased in patients with polycystic ovary syndrome (PCOS) andassociated with adiposity, but unaffected by pioglitazone treatment. Clin Endocrinol 2009; 71:652–58.

19. Niu J, Kolattukudy PE. Role of MCP-1 in cardiovascular disease: molecular mechanisms and clinical implications. Clin Sci (Lond) 2009; 117:95–109.

20. de Jager SC, Kraaijeveld AO, Grauss RW, de Jager W, Liem SS, van der Hoeven BL, et al. CCL3 (MIP-1 alpha) levels are elevated during acute coronary syndromes and show strong prognostic power for future ischemic events. J Mol Cell Cardiol 2008; 45:446–52.

21. Kebapcilar L, Taner CE, Kebapcilar AG, Sari I. High mean platelet volume, low-grade systemic coagulation and fibrinolytic activation are associated with androgen and insulin levels in polycystic ovary syndrome. Arch Gynecol Obstet 2009; 280:187–93.

22. Ruan X, Dai Y. Study on chronic low-grade inflammation and influentialfactors of polycystic ovary syndrome. Med Princ Pract 2009; 18:118–22.

23. Hulsmans M, Holvoet P. The vicious circle between oxidative stress and inflammation in atherosclerosis. J Cell Mol Med 2010; 14:70–78.

24. Barlovic DP, Thomas MC, Jandeleit-Dahm K. Cardiovascular disease: what's all theAGE/RAGE about? Cardiovasc Hematol Disord Drug Targets 2010; 10:7–15.

25. Low Grade Chronic Inflammation in Women with Polycystic Ovarian Syndrome Chris C. J. Kelly, Helen Lyall, John R. Petrie, Gwyn W. Gould, John M. C. Connell, Naveed Sattar The Journal of Clinical Endocrinology and Metabolism, Volume 86, Issue 6, 1 June 2001, Pages 2453–2455.

26. Parkes GC, Brostoff J, Whelan K, Sanderson JD. Gastrointestinal microbiota inirritable bowel syndrome: their role in its pathogenesis and treatment. Am J Gastroenterol 2008; 103(6):1557–67.

27. Maes M, Twisk FN, Kubera M, Ringel K. Evidence for inflammation and activation of cell-mediated immunity in myalgic encephalo-myelitis/chronic fatigue syndrome (ME/CFS): increased interleukin-1, tumor necrosis factora, PMN-elastase, lysozyme and neopterin. J Affect Disord 2011.

28. Kelton Tremellen, Karma Pearce. Dysbiosis of gut microbiota (DOGMA)–A novel theory for the development of Polycystic Ovarian Syndrome. Medical Hypotheses 2012; 79:104–112.

29. Wild RA, Painter PC, Coulson PB, Carruth KB, Ranney GB. Lipoprotein lipid concentrations and cardiovascular risk in women with polycystic ovary syndrome. J Clin Endocrinol Metab 1985; 61(5):946–51.

30. Barr S, Hart K, Reeves S, Sharp K, Jeanes YM. Habitual dietary intake, eating pattern and physical activity of women with polycystic ovary syndrome. Eur J ClinNutr 2011; 65(10):1126–32.

31. Cani PD, Amar J, Iglesias MA, et al. Metabolic endotoxemia initiates obesity and insulin resistance. Diabetes 2007; 56(7):1761–72.

32. Cani PD, Delzenne NM. Interplay between obesity and associated metabolic disorders: new insights into the gut microbiota. Curr Opin Pharmacol 2009; 9(6):737–43.

33. Wu GD, Chen J, Hoffmann C, et al. Linking long-term dietary patterns with gut microbial enterotypes. Science 2011; 334(6052):105–08.

34. Cani PD, Neyrinck AM, Fava F, et al. Selective increases of bifidobacteria in gutmicroflora improve high-fat-diet-induced diabetes in mice

through amechanism associated with endo-toxaemia. Diabetologia 2007; 50(11):2374–83.

35. Gummesson A, Carlsson LM, Storlien LH, et al. Intestinal permeability isassociated with visceral adiposity in healthy women. Obesity (Silver Spring) 2011; 19(11):2280–82.

36. Samsami DA, Razmjoei P, Parsanezhad ME. Serum levels of anti-histone and anti-double-strand DNA antibodies before and after laparo-scopic ovarian drilling in women with polycystic ovarian syndrome. Journal of Obstetrics and Gynecology of India 2014;64(1):47–52. doi: 10.1007/s13224-013-0451-x.

37. Samsami Dehaghani A, Karimaghaei N, Parsanezhad ME, Malekzadeh M, Mehrazmay M, Erfani N. Anti-nuclear antibodies in patients with polycystic ovary syndrome before and after laparoscopic electrocauterization. Iranian Journal of Medical Sciences 2013;38(2):187–90.

38. Cooper DS. Subclinical hypothyroidism. The New England Journal of Medicine 2001; 345(4):260–65. doi: 10.1056/nejm200107263450406.

39. Saravanan P, Dayan CM. Thyroid auto-antibodies. Endocrinology and Metabolism Clinics of North America. 2001;30(2):315–337. doi: 10.1016/s0889-8529(05)70189-4.

40. Petrikova J, Lazurova I, Dravecka I, et al. The prevalence of non organ specific and thyroid autoimmunity in patients with polycystic ovary syndrome. Biomedical Papers of the Medical Faculty of the University Palacky, Olomouc, Czechoslovakia. 2015;159(2):302–306. doi: 10.5507/bp.2014.062.

41. Janssen OE, Mehlmauer N, Hahn S, Öffner A H, Gärtner R. High prevalence of autoimmune thyroiditis in patients with polycystic ovary syndrome. European Journal of Endocrinology. 2004;150(3):363–69. doi: 10.1530/eje.0.1500363.

42. Kachuei M, Jafari F, Kachuei A, Keshteli AH. Prevalence of autoimmune thyroiditis in patients with polycystic ovary syndrome. Archives of Gynecology and Obstetrics 2012; 285(3):853–856. doi: 10.1007/s00404-011-2040-5.

43. Arduc A, Dogan BA, Bilmez S, et al. High prevalence of Hashimoto's thyroiditis in patients with polycystic ovary syndrome: does the imbalance between estradiol and progesterone play a role? Endocrine Research. 2015; 40(4):204–10. doi: 10.3109/07435800.2015.1015730.

44. Sarkar D. Recurrent pregnancy loss in patients with thyroid dysfunction. Indian Journal of Endocrinology and Metabolism 2012; 16(2): 350–51.

45. Lebovitz HE. Adjunct therapy for type 1 diabetes mellitus. Nature Reviews Endocrinology. 2010; 6(6):326–34. doi: 10.1038/nrendo.2010.49.

46. Gardener SG, Gale EAM, Williams AJK, et al. Progression to diabetes in relatives with islet autoantibodies. Is it inevitable? Diabetes Care. 1999; 22(12):2049–54.

HPO Axis and Metabolic Derangements in PCOS

Ashok Kumar, Divya KV

Polycystic ovarian syndrome (PCOS) is the most common endocrinopathy among women in reproductive age group characterised by significant metabolic abnormalities. Its prevalence is as high as 15% when diagnosed by Rotterdam criteria.[1] PCOS is characterized by a wide spectrum of signs and symptoms ranging from a single finding of polycystic ovarian morphology on ultrasound to obesity, hyperandrogenism, menstrual disturbances and insulin resistance. The clinical entity associated with polycystic ovaries is more regularly called syndrome due to its heterogeneous nature with more than one etiology. However, the exact cause of polycystic ovaries is unknown.[2] Involvement of two key genes in the etiology has been suggested, the steroid synthesis gene CYP11a and the insulin gene variable number tandem repeat. Familial clustering of PCOS cases suggests a major genetic component to its etiology with autosomal dominant inheritance.[3] Polycystic ovaries are characterized by defect at the hypothalamus, pituitary gland and ovary.

PITUITARY GONADOTROPINS

The pituitary gonadotropins have central role in reproductive function. The secretion of follicle-stimulating hormone (FSH) and luteinizing hormone is directly stimulated by hypothalamic gonadotropins and also influenced by the integrated feedback mechanism. Follicle-stimulating hormone provides initial stimulus for follicular development and also promotes granulosa cell conversion of androgen to estrogen by stimulating the aromatase enzyme. Luteinizing hormone is important in luteal phase by promoting progesterone secretion, also has a vital role in the follicular phase inducing thecal androgen production. Women with PCOS have an increased frequency of hypothalamic GnRH pulses, which in turn results in an increase in the LH/FSH ratio. The increased number of small follicles and their abnormal growth pattern are key features of PCOS. Hyperfunctioning of the thecal compartment with accumulation of multiple, small antral follicles, which are neither atretic nor apoptotic but arrested in development. Anti-müllerian hormone (AMH) levels progressively decrease as follicles increase in size. In women with PCOS, AMH levels are elevated and play an important role in long term disruption of ovarian physiology and elevated AMH levels are associated with infertility. Classic PCOS have a characteristic ovarian secretory response to gonadotropin stimulation, principally hyper-response to androstenedione secretion.

HYPERANDROGENISM

Hyperandrogenism is the most common feature of PCOS due to dysregulation of androgen secretion. The ovary is usually thought of the principal supply of androgens; however, several patients with PCOS even have multiplied adrenal steroid hormone secretion. It is possible that androgen hyper-responsivity is due to direct (via adrenocorticotropic hormone) or indirect (via corticotropin-releasing hormone) stimulation of the adrenal cortex. Increased urinary free cortisol has also been reported in PCOS patients. This alteration has been attributed to enhanced cortisol metabolism, followed by a compensatory overdrive of the hypothalamic-pituitary-adrenal axis and hence increased androgen production. An abnormal P450c17 function is principally responsible for the adrenal androgen excess in PCOS. Increased inactivation of cortisol by 5 β-reductase lowers cortisol blood levels and stimulates ACTH-dependent steroidogenesis.[4] Therefore, increased 5α-reductase or decreased 11β-hydroxysteroid dehydrogenase type 1 (11βHSD1) activity would enhance cortisol metabolism resulting in a compensatory increase in ACTH secretion and stimulation of adrenal steroidogenesis.[5–7]

Insulin disrupts all the components of the hypothalamus-pituitary-ovary axis results in impaired metabolic signaling resulting in hyperandrogenism. Insulin causes the liver to decrease production of a key molecule called sex hormone binding simple protein (SHBG). If a reduced quantity of SHBG is out there, a lot of free androgenic hormone is within the blood. It is additionally believed that prime levels of internal secretion will increase the quantity of androgens that the ovary produces. Androgens inturn lead to insulin resistance by increasing level of free fatty acids and modifying muscle tissue composition thus perpetuating hyperinsulinemia-hyperandrogenemia cycle.

OVARIAN STEROIDOGENESIS

Abnormal ovarian steroidogenesis seen in PCOS is due to intrinsic defects in ovary, particularly due to hypersecretion of luteinizing hormone (LH) and of insulin. Hypersecretion of LH is secondary to disturbance of nonsteroidal ovarian-pituitary feedback. Women with PCOS have reduced chances of conception and increased risk of miscarriage in those with elevated LH levels.

Women with PCOS are at increased risk for impaired glucose tolerance and type 2 diabetes.[8–10] In PCOS patients; β-cell activity is exaggerated leading to abnormality in insulin secretion. Aging causes beta cell failure, leading to glucose intolerance which may result in type 2 diabetes mellitus. Obesity, especially upper body obesity is a well known feature in PCOS and affects about 50% of patients. It has been studied that obese patients have significantly lower serum levels of sex hormone-binding globulin (SHBG) and high levels of free testosterone leading to hirsutism. Hyperinsulinemia is one of the contributing factors for hirsutism by reducing serum SHBG. Chronic anovulation seen in PCOS leads to menstrual abnormalities. PCOS is associated with deranged lipid profile and therefore is a definite risk factor for myocardial infarction. Amenorrheic women with PCO are at a risk of endometrial carcinoma and are generally associated with a favourable prognosis.[11] PCOS is associated with multiple metabolic derangements such as diabetes, hyperandrogenism, hirsutism, etc. and therefore, dietary modification with regular exercise is of paramount importance.

ALTERATIONS OF HPA AXIS ACTIVITY, INSULIN RESISTANCE, AND METABOLIC SYNDROME

It has been proposed that the metabolic abnormalities described in this syndrome are present before the onset of hyperandrogenism. Adiponectin is a 29-kDa adipocyte-derived protein that is involved in the regulation of insulin action and glucose metabolism. Serum adiponectin levels are inversely correlated with body mass index (BMI) and also with insulin resistance independent of BMI.[12,13] In adult women with PCOS, adiponectin concentrations change according to variations in fat mass and are apparently independent of insulin resistance.[14]

Some of the metabolic features of PCOS are present in daughters of PCOS women during childhood, well before the onset of hyperandrogenism. It has been observed that normal-weight prepubertal daughters of PCOS women exhibit significantly lower adiponectin concentrations, compared with daughters of normal women. This suggests that adiponectin concentrations could serve as an early marker of metabolic derangement in these girls, independent of body weight.[15]

Metabolic syndrome may be a constellation of metabolic disorders that embody primarily abdominal fatness, hypoglycemic agent resistance, impaired aldohexose metabolism, high blood pressure and dyslipidemia. It is understood that insulin resistance has a crucial pathophysiological role in the expression of all features of metabolic syndrome, particularly abdominal obesity.[16, 17] Coviello et al. reported that hyperandrogenemia is an important risk factor for metabolic syndrome in women with PCOS in addition to obesity and insulin resistance.[18] The interaction between insulin resistance, dyslipidemia, and hyperandrogenism in PCOS makes a vicious cycle, and highlights the timely diagnosis and treatment of PCOS.[19]

Glueck et al. reported that 46% of the women with PCOS had metabolic syndrome.[20] PCOS shares many clinical features with metabolic syndrome, including insulin resistance, obesity, type 2 diabetes mellitus (DM), hyperlipidemia, and hypertension. Among these characteristics, obesity is one amongst the foremost common options in women with PCOS. Approximately 50% of women with PCOS are overweight or obese.[21]

Epidemiologic studies have provided evidence for a significant positive association between cortisol levels and surrogate measures of insulin resistance or metabolic alterations, other than indices of overweight or obesity.[22–24] A mild cortisol increase was identified as an early feature of essential hypertension.[24] The cortisol blood levels may also represent an independent risk factor for CVDs, at least in South Asian individuals, suggesting that increased glucocorticoid action may contribute to ethnic differences in the prevalence of metabolic syndrome.[25] The metabolic alterations that occur in obesity and PCOS alter endometrial receptivity and thus likely affect proper embryonic implantation, resulting in increased miscarriage rates and overall subfertility.

In conclusion, female internal reproductive organ dysfunction is vital to the pathophysiology in polycystic ovary syndrome. Theca cells of PCOS patients have a generalised active steroidogenesis. The surplus sex hormone production from female reproductive organ or adrenals lead to inactive follicle development resulting in chronic oligo or anovulation. Hyperinsulinemia plays a very important role in the augmented sex hormone production. Basic pathology in PCOS affects the hypothalamic-pituitary-ovarian axis. As a consequence, PCOS is related to augmented risk of sterility, and in long run lead to pair of polygenic disorder and cardiovascular issues too.

REFERENCES

1. Fauser BC, Tarlatzis BC, Rebar RW, et al. agreement on women's health aspects of polycystic ovary syndrome (PCOS): the capital of The Netherlands ESHRE/ASRM-Sponsored third PCOS agreement Workshop cluster. Fertil Steril. 2012; 97(1):28–38. e25.
2. Han Y, Kim HS, Lee HJ, Oh JY, Sung YA. Metabolic effects of polycystic ovary syndrome in adolescents. Ann Pediatr Endocrinol Metab. 2015; 20(3):136–42.
3. Homburg R. Polycystic ovary syndrome: agreement and difference of opinion. 2001.
4. Gambineri A, Forlani G, Munarini A, et al. exaggerated clearance of adrenal cortical steroid by 5beta-reductase during a subgroup of ladies with adrenal hyperandrogenism in polycystic ovary syndrome. J Endocrinol Invest. 2009; 32(3):210–8.
5. Stewart PM, Shackleton CH, Beastall GH, Edwards CR. Five alpha-reductase activity in polycystic ovary syndrome. Lancet. 1990; 335:431–3.

6. Vassiliadi district attorney, Barber TM, Hughes BA, et al. exaggerated five alpha-reductase activity and cortex drive in girls with polycystic ovary syndrome. J Clin Endocrinol Metab. 2009; 94:3558–66.

7. Chin D, Shackleton C, Prasad VK, et al. exaggerated 5alpha-reductase and traditional 11beta-hydroxysteroid dehydrogenase metabolism of C19 and C21 steroids during a young population with polycystic gonad syndrome. J Pediatr Endocrinol Metab. 2000; 13:253–9.

8. Ehrmann DA, Barnes RB, Rosenfield RL, Cavaghan MK, Imperial J. Prevalence of impaired aldohexose tolerance and polygenic disease in girls with polycystic ovary syndrome. polygenic disease Care. 1999; 22:141–6.

9. Legro RS, Kunselman AR, Dodson WC, Dunaif A. Prevalence and predictors of risk for sort II diabetes and impaired aldohexose tolerance in polycystic ovary syndrome: a prospective, controlled study in 254 affected girls. J Clin Endocrinol Metab 1999; 84:165–9.

10. O'Meara NM, Blackman JD, Ehrmann DA. Defects in β-cell function in functional ovarian hyperandrogenism. J Clin Endocrinol Metab. 1993; 76:1241–7.

11. Rojas J, Chávez M, Olivar L, et al. Polycystic ovary syndrome, hormone resistance, and obesity: navigating the pathophysiologic labyrinth. Int J Reprod MEd. 2014; 2014:719050.

12. Arita Y, Kihara S, Ouchi N, et al. Incomprehensible decrease of associate adipose-specific supermolecule, adiponectin, in obesity. Biochem Biophys Res Commun. 1999; 2:79–83.

13. Weyer C, Funahashi T, Tanaka S, et al. Hypoadiponectinemia in fat and sort a pair of diabetes: shut association with hormone resistance and hyperinsulinemia. J Clin Endocrinol Metab. 2001; 86:1930–5.

14. Orio Jr F, Palomba S, Cascella T, et al. Adiponectin levels in girls with polycystic ovary syndrome. J Clin Endocrinol Metab. 2003; 88:2619–23.

15. Sir-Petermann T, Maliqueo M, Codner E, et al. Early metabolic derangements in daughters of ladies with polycystic ovary syndrome. J Clin Endocrinol Metab. 2007 Dec;92(12):4637–42.

16. Reaven GM. hormone resistance in human malady. Diabetes. 1988; 37:1595–607.

17. Phillips DI, Barker DJ, Fall CH, et al. Elevated plasma adrenal cortical steroid concentrations: a link between low birth weight and also the hormone resistance syndrome? J. Clin. Endocrinol. Metab. 1998; 83:757–60.

18. Coviello AD, Legro RS, Dunaif A. Adolescent ladies with polycystic ovary syndrome have associate exaggerated risk of the metabolic syndrome related to increasing steroid hormone levels freelance of fat and hormone resistance. J Clin Endocrinol Metab. 2006; 91:492–7.

19. Sozen I, Arici A. Hyperinsulinism and its interaction with hyperandrogenism in polycystic ovary syndrome. Obstet Gynecol Surv. 2000; 55:321–8.

20. Glueck CJ, Papanna R, Wang P, Goldenberg N, Sieve-Smith L. Incidence and treatment of metabolic syndrome in fresh referred girls with confirmed polycystic gonad syndrome. Metabolism. 2003; 52:908–15.

21. Pasquali R, Casimirri F. The impact of fat on hyperandrogenism and polycystic ovary syndrome in biological time girls. Clin Endocrinol (Oxf.) 1993; 39:1–16.

22. Phillips DI, Barker DJ, Fall CH, et al. Elevated plasma adrenal cortical steroid concentrations: a link between low birth weight and also the hormone resistance syndrome? J Clin Endocrinol Metab. 1998; 83:757–60.

23. Dinneen S, Alzaid A, Miles J, Rizza R. Metabolic effects of the nocturnal rise in adrenal cortical steroid on macromolecule metabolism in traditional humans. J Clin Invest 1993; 92:2283–90.

24. Walker BR, Phillips DI, Noon JP, et al. Exaggerated hormone activity in men with vessel risk factors. High Blood Pressure. 1998; 31:891–5.

25. Ward AM, Fall CH, Stein CE, et al. Adrenal cortical steroid and also the metabolic syndrome in South Asians. Clin. Endocrinol (Oxf). 2003; 58:500–5.

5

Hyperandrogenism and PCOS

Suman Mittal, Anjali Deshpande

Androgen excess (AE) or hyperandrogenism is an endocrine disorder of reproductive age group. Excess androgen production is from ovary and adrenal glands. Hyperandrogenism is characterized by laboratory finding of an abnormally elevated serum concentration of androgen and/or the physical findings consistent with androgen excess. The most common conditions associated with hyperandrogenism are polycystic ovary syndrome (PCOS), a set of symptoms caused by androgen excess in females, and various cancers that can cause androgen excess.

Androgen Physiology and Pathophysiology

Androgens are intrinsic to the maintenance of ovarian and sexual function. Before exploring hyperandrogenic states, we must be knowledgeable with regard to the role of androgens and their interplay in the physiology of the women.

Androgens and their Effects

Androgens circulate in various forms. The majority of circulating androgens found in the blood of premenopausal women are in the form of androstenedione and testosterone. Androstenedione circulates bound to both sex hormone-binding globulin (SHBG) and albumin.

Under normal circumstances, the ovaries and adrenal glands contribute nearly equal to testosterone production.

Approximately 25% of circulating testosterone is derived from the ovary; an equal proportion is of adrenal origin. The remaining 50% of testosterone in the circulation is derived from the conversion of androstenedione, which in tern equally contributed to by the adrenal and ovary. The majority of DHEA is of adrenal origin; 50% is directly secreted, and 30% is derived from conversion of DHEAS. A small proportion (20%) of circulating DHEA comes from ovarian secretion. Finally, DHEAS is almost entirely derived from direct secretion by the adrenal.

Hyperandrogenism and PCOS

Androgen excess (AE), an essential feature of the polycystic ovary syndrome, is primarily

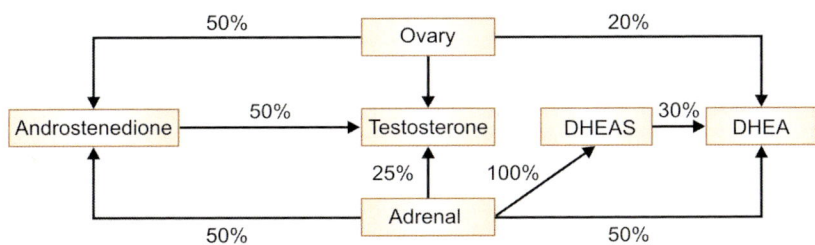

Fig. 5.1: Flowchart depicting source of androgen production

ovarian origin, although a hyperactivity of adrenocortical function of adrenal androgen (AA) excess is present in a significant number of patients.

Key Points for AE in PCOS

1. ↑ Ovarian theca cell function.
2. ↑ Expression of steroidogenic enzymes.
3. ↑ LH stimulation of thecal androgen bio-synthesis.
4. Abnormalities in intrinsic ovarian factors such as inhibin, activin, and follistatin appear to modulate ovarian LH response.
5. Granulosa cell dysfunction.

Clinical Observation

These hyperandrogenic features impact considerably on quality of life in women with PCOS. Symptoms of hyperandrogenism depend upon degree of androgenism.

1. Non-virilizing symptoms
2. Virilizing symptoms

1. *Non-Virilizing Symptoms*

a. Hirsutism
b. Acne

2. *Virilizing Symptoms*

a. Alopecia
b. Deepening of voice
c. Musculinization of body
d. Clitoromegaly
e. Increase libido

Hirsutism

The most recognizable clinical sign of hyperandrogenism is hirsutism. Hirsutism refers to growth of dark terminal hair on the face, chest, back, lower abdomen, and upper thighs caused by overactivity of circulating androgen hormones. Androgen stimulates hair growth, increases the diameter of hair shaft, and deepen the pigmentation of hair. Elevated androgens are detected in the vast majority (>70%) of women with hirsutism. The most common

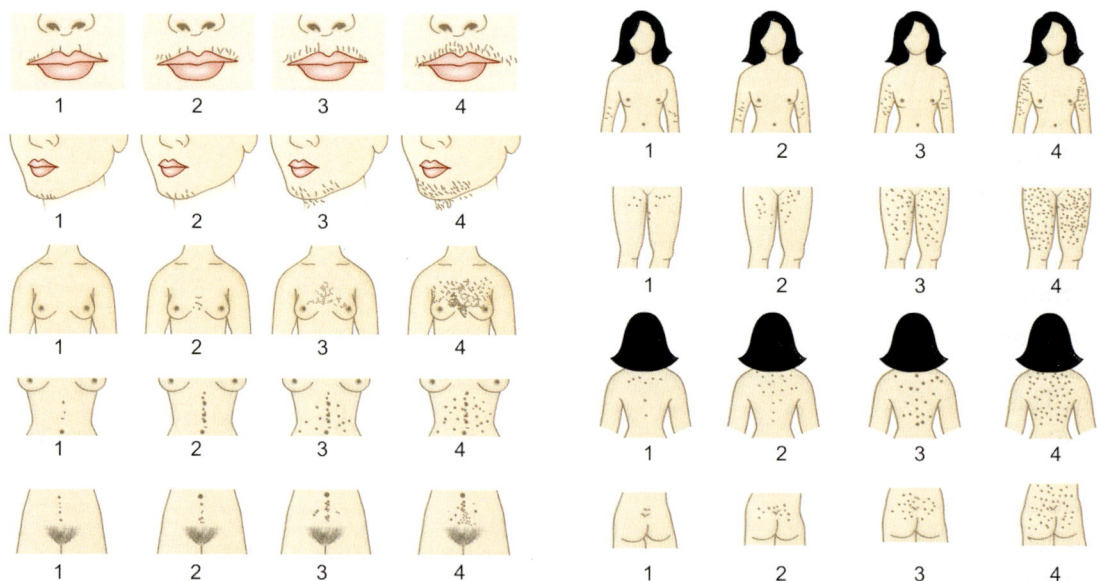

Fig. 5.2: The Ferriman-Gallwey scoring system for hirsutism. (Reprinted from Hatch R Rosenfield RL, Kim MH. Tredway D Hirsustism: implications, etiology, and management. Am J Obstet. Gynecol. 1981:140: B15. Copyright 1981, with permission from Elsevier

visual assessment tool is the modified Ferriman-Gallwey score.[2,3]

Nine body areas are graded from 0 (no terminal hair) to 4 (Frankly vinile) and the sum totaled. Level ≥4–6 indicates hirsutism, which is ethnicity dependent. If vellus and terminal hairs are not distinguished, hirsutism may be over-estimated. Only terminal hairs need to be considered in pathological hirsutism, with terminal hairs clinically growing >5 mm in length if untreated, varying in shape and texture and generally being pigmented.

Acne

Common disorder of pilosebaceous unit (PSU) androgen excess causes excessive secretion of sebum. Lesion of the PSU called acne. Acne is associated with biochemical hyperandrogenism,[4,5] yet the predictive value of acne alone is unclear[1,4] and there is no accepted assessment tool.[1]

Alopecia

It is recession of frontal hair, as well as loss of hair in the temporal regions of the scalp and the crown of the head in response to androgens. Most studies of women with alopecia reveal a relatively low prevalence of hyperandrogenemia.[1,6] The predictive value of alopecia is unclear due to multiple etiologies. Hair loss on the scalp is usually assessed visually using the Ludwig scale.[1]

Deepening of Voice

In response to excessive androgen exposure, vocal cord undergoes an irreversible thickening. This results in lowering the tone of the voice.

Musculinization of Body

Hypertrophy of major muscle groups, such as arm and leg muscles, occurs in response to androgen exposure. Muscle cells become larger, and there number increases as well. Hypertrophy of major muscle groups result in the development of what is commonly described as a male body habitus.

Clitoromegaly

Enlargement of the clitoris may occur in response to excessive androgen exposure. This is dose-dependent event and irreversible.

Causes of Hyperandrogenism

1. Polycystic ovary syndrome
2. Idiopathic hirsutism
3. Hyperandrogenic insulin resistant acanthosis nigricans (HAIR-AN) syndrome
4. Congenital adrenal hyperplasia
5. Cushing syndrome
6. Androgen-secreting tumors (ovarian, adrenal)
7. Hyperprolactenemia
8. Hypothyroidism
9. Androgenic medication (e.g. danazol)

Biochemical Evolution of Hyperandrogenemia

1. ***Total and free testosterone:*** Assessment of biochemical hyperandrogenism is most useful in establishing the diagnosis of PCOS and/or phenotype where clinical signs of hyperandrogenism (in particular hirsutism) are unclear or absent.
   - Testosterone is the key androgen to measure. However, the sensitivity and specificity of methods for directly assessing total circulating testosterone levels (e.g. direct radioimmunoassays or chemiluminescence immunoassays) is less.
   - No reliable direct assays for total or free testosterone assessment are available currently. However, the amount of bio-available testosterone, calculated free testosterone, or free androgen index (FAI) can be calculated.
   - For precise assessment of total or free testosterone in PCOS, high quality assays such as liquid chromatography-mass

spectrometry (LCMS)/mass spectrometry and extraction/chromatography immuno-assays, may be used. Testosterone secretion may be increased during mid-cycle and assessment of androgen status should preferably be during the early follicular phase (D 4–10) in normally cycling women, whilst diurnal variation means morning levels may be most predictive.

- Where androgen levels are markedly above laboratory reference ranges, (>200 ng/mL) other causes of biochemical hyperandrogenism (neoplasm) need to be considered.
- In women on hormonal contraception, reliable assessment of biochemical hyperandrogenism is not possible due to effects on sex hormone-binding globulin and altered gonadotropin-dependent androgen production. In such cases, drug withdrawal is recommended for 3 months or longer before measurement.

2. *Other androgen (androstenedione and DHEAS):* It is of little use in most patients. Androstenedione and dehydroepiandro-sterone sulfate (DHEAS) could be considered if total or free testosterones are not elevated; however, these provide limited additional information in the diagnosis of PCOS. It is increased in approximate 15% of women who have normal total and free testosterone levels.

Once hyperandrogenemia is documented, the diagnosis of PCOS is made when other hyperandrogenic disorders are excluded. We need following tests to exclude these.

3. *Tests exclude other causes of hyperandro-genism*
   a. 17-alpha hydroxyprogesteron (17-OHP)-100–300 ng/dL is normal range
   b. Thyroid function test
   c. Serum prolactin
   d. Insulin function test
   e. USG

TABLE 5.1: Differential diagnosis of hyperandrogenism

Diagnosis	Incidence	Additional findings	Testing
Polycystic ovary syndrome	82%	Irregular menses, glucose intolerance, elevated blood pressure	Elevated insulin levels, multiple ovarian cysts on ultrasound
Hyperandrogenism with normal ovulation	7%	Regular menses	Elevated androgen levels
Idiopathic hirsutism	5%	Regular menses	Normal androgen levels
Hyperandrogenic insulin-resistant acanthosis nigricans (HAIRAN)	3%	Acanthosis nigricans	Elevated fasting glucose and insulin levels
Late-onset congenital adrenal hyperplasia (non-classic)	2%	Short stature	Elevated 17-OH-progesterone
Congenital adrenal hyperplasia (21-hydroxylase deficiency)	1%	Possible virilization	Elevated 17-OH-progesterone
Hypothyroidism	<1%	Fatigue, weight gain, amenorrhea	Elevated thyroid-stimulating hormone, low free thyroxine
Hyperprolactinemia	<1%	Amenorrhea, galactorrhea, fertility	Elevated prolactin levels
Androgen-secreting neoplasm	<1%	Rapid-onset hirsutism	Mass seen on pelvic ultrasound, abdominal computed tomography
Cushing's syndrome	<1%	Abdominal striae, central obesity	Elevated cortisol levels

Treatment

Treatment of hyperandrogenism is sought for:

- Reduction of hair growth
- Reduction of acne
- Restoration of menstrual cycle
- Infertility
- Metabolic abnormalities

A problem-oriented approach to the treatment of patient with androgen excess follows:

1. Lifestyle modification and weight reduction
2. Cosmetic
3. Pharmacological treatments

1. *Lifestyle modification:* This is the first line of PCOS management. Healthy lifestyle including healthy eating and regular exercise is recommended in all cases of PCOS to achieve and maintain healthy weight and to optimize hormonal outcomes, and quality of life. Lifestyle intervention preferably multicomponent including:
   a. Diet
   b. Exercise
   c. Behavioural strategies

   Weight loss of as little as 5–10% has been demonstrated to correct hyperandrogenism, menstrual irregularities and insulin resistance.

2. *Cosmetic:* It includes:
   a. Epilation methods
   b. Electrolysis
   c. Laser

   a. *Epilation methods:* Most women resort to removal of hair by different epilation methods such as plucking, shaving, and waxing before presenting to the clinic. Though these methods are simple, inexpensive and temporary, their side-effects include physical discomfort, scarring, folliculitis, irritant dermatitis or discoloration.

   b. *Electrolysis:* Electrolysis has also been used for the removal of the hair. With repeated treatments, the efficacy ranges from 15 to 50% permanent hair loss[7] However, it is difficult to treat large areas like hairs on the chest or upper back with electrolysis and it can be time consuming.

   c. *Laser:* Laser has gained wide popularity in past two decades and can achieve permanent reduction of hair, not removal. They work on the principle of selective photothermolysis where the laser energy acts specifically to destroy the target (melanin).[8,9] Laser energy acts on only anagen hair follicles. Therefore, multiple treatments are required to get a significant reduction. An ideal candidate for laser hair removal is a patient with light skin color and dark-colored hairs. Different lasers for hair removal include 694 nm ruby laser, the 1064 nm Q-switched Nd:YAG laser, the 755 nm long-pulsed alexandrite, and the 800 nm diode laser. For Indian skin types (type IV and V), long wavelength lasers like the Nd:YAG laser have been found to be most effective.[10]

3. *Pharmacological treatment:* Medical treatment of acne and hirsutism despite cosmetic measures involve reduction of androgen levels and their effect on their end organ effect. This is usually accomplished by:
   a. Suppression of ovarian androgen production
   b. Alteration of binding of androgens to their plasma binding protein
   c. Impairment of peripheral conversion of androgen precursors to active androgen.
   d. Inhibition of androgen action at target tissue level.

The following drugs can be used:

1. Oral contraceptives
2. Antiandrogen:
   a. Spironolactone
   b. Cyproteron acetate
   c. Finasteride
   d. Flutamide

1. Oral Contraceptives

Oral contraceptives are considered first-line for treating hirsutism, particularly in those women who are desirous of contraception. Estrogen/progesterone combinations act by-

a. Reducing gonadotropin secretion and thereby reducing ovarian androgen production.[11]

b. Increasing levels of SHBG resulting in lower levels of free testosterone.

c. Inhibiting adrenal androgen production.[12]

However there is no clinical evidence that any one oral contraceptive is superior to another.[13] Assessment of adequacy of androgen suppression can be made at the end of third week after starting treatment.[14] The effect on acne can be expected to be maximal in 1–2 months. In contrast, the effect on hair growth may not be evident for 6 months and the maximum effect requires 9–12 months.

2. Antiandrogen

a. *Spironolactone:* Spironolactone is an androgen blocker and competes with DHT for binding to the androgen receptor. It has a variable progestational activity and reduces the production of ovarian androgens. Its beneficial effects take at least 6 months to show. Side effects include polyuria, and hypotension with associated headaches, fatigue, or even syncope.

b. *Cyproterone acetate:* Cyproterone acetate has strong progestogenic and antiandrogen properties. It produces a decrease in circulating testosterone and androstenedione levels through a reduction in circulating LH and has been used as an effective treatment for hirsutism.[15] CPA is commercially available in combination with ethinyl estradiol (2 mg CPA and 35 µg EE/tablet).

c. *Finasteride:* Finasteride is a 5-α reductase inhibtor has been found to be effective in the treatment of hirsutism.[16] All these 5-RA agents have the potential of feminizing a male fetus. Hence, effective contraception must be used by patients on these drugs.

d. *Flutamide:* Flutamide is a potent non-steroidal antiandrogen without progestational, estrogenic, corticoid, androgenic activity[17] that appears to be efficacious in the treatment of hirsutism.[18] Dose is 250 mg twice daily. In a 7-month trial of flutamide in conjunction with OCPs, marked improvement in acne, seborrhea and hirsutism was reported.[19]

Current Research and Future Perspective

- Association of biochemical hyperandrogenism with type II diabetes mellitus and obesity in Chinese women with polycystic ovary syndrome.
- Genetic basis for hyperandrogenemia in polycystic ovarian syndrome.
- Genetic variants associated with hyperandrogenemia in PCOS pathophysiology.

CONCLUSION

In patients presenting with signs and symptoms of hyperandrogenism, a careful history, including time of onset (gradual or rapid), is critical. Rapid onset of hirsutism or virilization suggests an androgen-secreting tumor, whereas gradual onset of symptoms at puberty suggests PCOS, the most common underlying cause of hirsutism. If history and physical examination do not delineate the underlying cause, laboratory testing that includes measurement of total serum testosterone and DHEAS can be helpful. Oral contraceptives are the most widely used drugs for suppressing ovarian androgen production in women with hirsutism; however, more specific therapy is warranted in some diseases.

REFERENCES

1. Lizneva D, et al., Androgen excess: Investigations and management. Best Pract Res Clin Obstet Gynaecol. 2016; 37:98–118.

2. Ferriman D and JD Gallwey, Clinical assessment of body hair growth in women. J Clin Endocrinol Metab. 1961; 21:1440–7.

3. Yildiz BO, et al., Visually scoring hirsutism. Hum Reprod Update. 2010; 16(1):51–64.

4. Uysal G, et al., Is acne a sign of androgen excess disorder or not? Eur J Obstet Gynecol Reprod Biol. 2017; 211:21–5.

5. Slayden SM, et al., Hyperandrogenemia in patients presenting with acne. Fertil Steril. 2001; 75(5):889–92.

6. Olsen, E.A., et al., Evaluation and treatment of male and female pattern hair loss. J Am Acad Dermatol. 2005; 52(2):301–11.

7. Wagner RF, Jr Physical methods for the management of hirsutism. Cutis. 1990; 45:19–26.

8. Dierickx CC. Hair removal by lasers and intense pulsed light sources. Semin Cutan Med Surg. 2000;19:267–75.

9. Sanchez LA, Perez M, Azziz R. Laser hair reduction in the hirsute patient: A critical assessment. Hum Reprod Update. 2002;8:169–81.

10. Battle EF, Jr, Hobbs LM. Laser-assisted hair removal for darker skin types. Dermatol Ther. 2004;17:177–83.

11. Burkman RT, Jr. The role of oral contraceptives in the treatment of hyperandrogenic disorders. Am J Med. 1995; 98:130–6.

12. Shaw JC. Spironolactone in dermatological therapy. J Am Acad Dermatol. 1991; 24:236–43.

13. Martin KA, Chang RJ, Ehrmann DA, et al: Evaluation and treatment of hirsutism in premenopausal women.: an endocrine society clinical practice guideline, J Clin Endocrinol Metab 2008; 93(4):1105–20.

14. Givens J, Anderson R, Wiser W. Dynamics of suppression and recovery of plasma FSH,LH, androstenedione and testosterone in polycystic ovarian disease using an oral contraceptives. J Clin Endocrinol Metab. 1974; 38:727–35.

15. van der Spuy ZM, le Roux PA. Cyproterone acetate for hirsutism. Cochrane Database Syst Rev. 2003. CD001125.

16. Faloia E, Filipponi S, Mancini V, Di Marco S, Mantero F. Effect of finasteride in idiopathic hirsutism. J Endocrinol Invest. 1998; 21:694–8.

17. Neri R, Monahan M: Effects of a novel nonsteroidal antiandrogen on canine prostatic hyperplasia, Invest Urol. 1972; 10:123–30.

18. Swiglo BA, Cosma M, Flynn DN, et al. Clinical review: Antiandrogens for the treatment of hirsutism: A systemic review and metaanalysis of randamised control trials. J Clin Endocrinol Metab. 2008; 93(4):1153–60.

19. Cusan L, Dupont A, Belanger A, et al: Treatment of hirsutism with the pure antiandrogen flutamide, J Am Acad Dermatol. 1990; 23:462–469.

Lipotoxicity and Insulin Resistance in PCOS

Smiti Nanda, Anjali Gupta

PCOS (polycystic ovarian syndrome) is a major endocrinopathy affecting 6–10% of reproductive age women.[1] It is characterized by chronic anovulation, hyperandrogenism and polycystic ovaries. Recent research trials suggest that PCOS is associated with metabolic complications including obesity, insulin resistance, type 2 diabetes mellitus, hypertension, dyslipidemia, metabolic syndrome, nonalcoholic fatty liver disease and cardiovascular disease.[2]

Pathophysiology

Its pathogenesis is still unclear. Insulin resistance has been reported consistently among many women having PCOS , especially in women having hyperandrogenism.[3]

What is Insulin Resistance?

Insulin resistance is classically defined as the reduced ability of insulin to stimulate glucose disappearance in peripheral tissues as well as inhibits hepatic glucose production and adipose tissue lipolysis which corresponds to the main metabolic actions of insulin.[4] This leads to increase in the level of glucose in the blood. This may cause rise in insulin production as the body tries to move glucose into cells. Insulin resistance increases the risk of type 2 diabetes and cardiovascular disease and these factors should be considered when determining long-term treatment.[5]

Insulin Signalling Pathways in Women with PCOS

Majority studies in women with PCOS were performed on muscle, adipose tissues, and also on fibroblasts that are easily accessible and insulin sensitive tissues. In fibroblast and muscle cells, it was found that serine phosphorylation of the insulin receptor or insulin receptor substrate-1 (IRS-1) is constitutively increased in PCOS women which was associated with a reduction in tyrosine phosphorylation of the insulin receptor and IRS and reduced PI3K activity. It was demonstrated in type 2 diabetes that signal transduction of the metabolic pathway of insulin is reduced when insulin receptors and IRS-1 or IRS-2 are serine-phosphorylated instead of tyrosine-phosphorylated. Study performed in muscular biopsies obtained during *in vivo* insulin infusion in PCOS women established altered association between IRS-1 and PI3K, which was correlated with reduced *in vivo* glucose uptake. Defective metabolic actions of insulin in PCOS women seem to involve initial insulin signaling steps and most likely result from abnormal serine phosphorylation rather than from defective protein express.[4]

It has been demonstrated that early steps in insulin signalling (maximal rate of glucose uptake, abundance of GLUT4, inhibition of lipolysis stimulated by insulin) were all decreased in PCOS women compared to controls, even if the number and affinity of insulin receptors are not obviously decreased in adipocytes from obese PCOS women. These findings were also observed in PCOS women presenting no obesity, glucose intolerance, or increased waist-to-hip ratio, suggesting that they may be intrinsic to the syndrome.[6]

Insulin Resistance and Hyperandrogenism

Hyperandrogenism, may have multiple causes, some not related to insulin resistance.

Studies have shown that women with PCOS display both adrenal and ovarian androgenic hyper-responsiveness to LH and ACTH. Interestingly, many studies found that this exaggerated androgenic response was curbed after treatment improving metabolic insulin resistance in both lean and obese PCOS women, but not after chronic suppression of LH or ACTH. These findings suggest that this hyper-responsiveness is not due to chronic LH or ACTH activation, but maybe caused by insulin resistance or related factors.[4]

A link between insulin and androgen production has been shown by many studies, Nestler et al. were the first to show that insulin levels were directly related to androgen production in vivo.[7] It has been demonstrated that with diazoxide, which reduces insulin secretion directly in pancreatic β-cells, lowered significantly free and total testosterone level in obese and hyperinsulinemic PCOS women.[8]

Androgen production is driven by two main enzymes—3β-hydroxysteroid dehydrogenase and P450c17 cytochrome, activities of which are increased in PCOS women. P450c17 enzyme exhibits 17α-hydroxylase and 17, 20-lyase activities, which are involved in the generation of two androgen precursors, dehydroepiandrosterone (DHEA) and andronestenedione. This lyase activity is favoured by serine/threonine phosphorylation of P450c17. Insulin may also stimulate P450c17 activity.[6,9]

Impairment in insulin signalling may be implicated in androgen overproduction at the level of androgen producing organs. Ovarian theca-interstitial cells express the enzyme P45017.[4]

A double blind placebo controlled study also demonstrated that lowering postprandial insulin levels, using acarbose slows down intestinal glucose absorption, significantly decreases the free androgen index among obese hyperinsulinemic PCOS women, in comparison to the placebo.[10] Moreover, it has been demonstrated that in lean normo-insulinemic PCOS women who were not insulin resistant, that lowering their insulin secretion with diazoxide for 8 days was associated with significantly decreased androgen levels and increased SHBG levels.[11]

It is emphasized that in healthy women, inhibition of insulin secretion with diazoxide does not have any effect on their testosterone levels. Accordingly, insulin does not seem to be related to androgen production in normal women, suggesting that androgenic hyper-responsiveness to insulin is specific to PCOS.[6]

Hyperinsulinemia directly reduces liver production of sex hormone-binding globulin (SHBG) levels, which acts as a testosterone carrier in plasma and thus lowers free testosterone levels, in obese women with the polycystic ovary syndrome independently of any effect on serum sex steroids.[12]

Despite the evidences in literature, the exact roles of insulin resistance and associated compensatory hyperinsulinemia for hyper-androgenism of PCOS are still debated.

Hyperinsulinemia associated with insulin resistance to explain PCOS hyperandrogenism, is probably not the main factor, because: (1) some women with PCOS have normal insulin sensitivity and are normoinsulinemic, and (2) most women with insulin resistance, due to obesity do not develop PCOS or hyperandrogenemia.

Recently lipotoxicity has been postulated critical in the development of PCOS causing hyperandrogenism and insulin resistance.

LIPOTOXICITY

Lipotoxicity is implicated in PCOS pathophysiology, both through increased androgen production and through induction of systemic insulin resistance.

Lipotoxicity literally means fat toxicity. It is a metabolic syndrome that results from the accumulation of lipid intermediates in non-adipose tissue, leading to cellular dysfunction and death. Normally in cellular operations, there is a balance between the production of lipids, and their oxidation or transport; however in lipotoxic cells, the balance between the amount of lipids produced and the amount used is disturbed.[13]

Adipocytes, handle the excess lipids in the body. When excess lipids overburden these cells, they start to leak their contents out into the blood, including fatty acids, leptin and other chemical messengers. When NEFAS (non-esterified fatty acids) leak from fat cells, cause a spill over into non-adipose cells, which do not have the necessary storage space cellular dysfunction and/or death results. This causes the cells to respond to insulin- and makes them insulin resistant. The cause of apoptosis and extent of cellular dysfunction is related to the type of cell affected, as well as the type and quantity of excess lipids.

Cellular NEFAs originate either from circulating NEFA or from triglycerides carried in the circulation by triglyceride-rich lipoproteins (chylomicrons and VLDL), which release NEFA under the action of lipoprotein lipase. Normal intracellular NEFA metabolism could be exceeded or impaired, in association with a genetic defect in mitochondrial β-oxidation in offspring of subjects with type 2 diabetes. In regard to intracellular mechanisms of lipotoxicity, it was observed that excessive mitochondrial NEFA β-oxidation may lead to the formation of reactive lipids, such as diacylglycerol (DAG) and ceramides. These mediators activate the serine/threonine kinase cascade leading to serine phosphorylation of the insulin receptor and insulin receptor substrates (IRS-1/2), causing a decrease in PI3K activation.[4] As for NEFA metabolites, the inflammation marker TNF-α is known to serine phosphorylate IRS-1, thus contributing to insulin resistance.[14]

It has been reported that lipid-overloaded hypertrophic adipocytes are insulin resistant independent of adipocyte inflammation associated with defect in glucose transporter 4 (GLUT4) trafficking to the plasma membrane. Very recently, it has been reported that early B cell factor 1 (EBF1) reduction caused adipocyte hypertrophy and insulin resistance but did not influence the inflammatory pathways in both mouse and human adipocytes.[15]

Overexposure of androgen-secreting tissues to NEFA and/or defective NEFA metabolism, leading to lipotoxic effects may induce androgen biosynthesis. Indeed, lipotoxicity could trigger androgenic hyper-responsiveness to insulin, LH, and ACTH. In most PCOS women, lipotoxicity also causes insulin resistance, inducing compensatory hyper-insulinemia, and may thus further increase hyperandrogenemia.[4]

NEFA-induced lipotoxicity may explain both the hyperandrogenemia and insulin resistance that characterize PCOS women. PPAR-γ agonists treatment which reduces lipotoxicity, improves systemic and cellular metabolism of NEFA and has been shown to treat PCOS hyperandrogenemia. Furthermore, recently AT2R activation is also able to improve lipotoxicity. AT2R signalling improves adipocyte size and nonadipose tissue NEFA uptake and might therefore prevent lipotoxicity and insulin resistance.[16]

Women would be predisposed to PCOS if their androgenic tissues are not able to appropriately metabolize NEFA or are too sensitive to the lipotoxic effects of NEFA, which could be acquired through genetic, epigenetic, or other developmental origins. With this predisposition, women who develop a more lipotoxic environment (increased circulating levels of NEFA or triglycerides) and/or insulin resistance with compensatory hyperinsulinemia, following weight gain or sedentary, for example, would display or exacerbate PCOS manifestations.[1]

Molecular Biology in Lipotoxicity causing Hyperandrogenism

Extracellular signal-regulated kinases (ERK), 1/2 component of mitogen-activated protein kinases (MAPK) pathway was shown to reduce by 50% in PCOS thecal cells whereas mitogen/extracellular signal-regulated kinase (MEK), 1/2 another component of MAPK was reduced by 70%. This is associated with increased androgen biosynthesis. Reduction in MEK/ERK pathway in PCOS women might overexpress the machinery of androgen biosynthesis which is further stimulated by LH, ACTH and insulin whereas origin of MEK/ERK pathway inhibition is the adverse intracellular consequence of NEFA.[16] Bellanger, et al. demonstrated that lipotoxicity through inhibition of MEK/ERK pathway can directly trigger androgen production in vitro.[17]

Lipotoxicity and Infertility

Lipotoxicity has been found to cause infertility. High follicular fluid NEFA levels were found to be correlated with poor oocyte quality and morphology in women undergoing *in vitro* fertilization. It was found that testosterone levels, measured in the ovarian follicular fluid, were positively associated with follicular fluid levels of lipids. Testosterone levels are negatively correlated with percentage of fertilized oocytes.[18]

Evaluation for Patients with Polycystic Ovary Syndrome for Insulin Resistance

All women with PCOS should be evaluated for signs of insulin resistance, type 2 diabetes and cardiovascular disease.

- Signs of insulin resistance-hypertension, obesity, centripetal fat distribution, and the presence of acanthosis nigricans. Acanthosis nigricans, noted on the back of the neck, in the axillae, underneath the breasts, and even on the vulva, is marked by velvety, mossy, verrucous, hyperpigmented skin. The presence of acanthosis nigricans appears to be more a sign of insulin resistance or medication reaction than a distinct disease itself. Other pathologic conditions such as insulinoma and adenocarcinoma of the stomach, may be rarely associated with acanthosis nigricans.

- Assess CVD risk (by assessing individual CVD risk factors (obesity, lack of physical activity, cigarette smoking, family history of type 2 diabetes, dyslipidaemia, hypertension, impaired glucose tolerance, type 2 diabetes) at baseline.

- Measure BMI and waist circumference (value greater than 35 inches = abnormal).

- Blood pressure (checked at the time of initial diagnosis and during oral contraceptive therapy). Drug therapy is considered for blood pressures greater than or equal to 140 mm Hg systolic and/or 90 mm Hg diastolic, not responding to lifestyle measures, (or diabetic patients or other high-risk factors with blood pressure greater than 130 mm Hg systolic and/or 80 mmHg diastolic).

- Women with a diagnosis of PCOS should be screened for type 2 diabetes and impaired glucose tolerance with a fasting glucose level followed by a 2-hour glucose level after a 75 g glucose load. 2-hour oral glucose tolerance test (fasting glucose less than 110 mg/dL = normal, 110–125 mg/dL = impaired, greater than 126 mg/dL = type 2 diabetes) followed by 75 g oral glucose ingestion and then 2-hour glucose level (less than 140 mg/dL = normal glucose tolerance, 140–199 mg/dL = impaired glucose tolerance, greater than 200 mg/dL = type 2 diabetes).

- In women with impaired fasting glucose (fasting plasma glucose level from 6.1 to

6.9 mmol/L) or impaired glucose tolerance (plasma glucose of 7.8 mmol/L or more but less than 11.1 mmol/L after a 2-hour oral glucose tolerance test), an oral glucose tolerance test should be performed annually.[19]

Management

Lifestyle Modification

Recommendation is that lifestyle changes (including diet, exercise and weight loss), should be considered as the first line of treatment in women with PCOS for improvement of long-term outcomes. These measures should precede and/or accompany the pharmacological treatment. In overweight women with PCOS, a reduction of as little as 5% of total body weight has been shown to reduce insulin resistance, testosterone levels and improvement in body composition and cardiovascular risk markers.[19]

Lifestyle management targeting weight loss (in women with a BMI of ≥ 25 kg/m^2) and prevention of weight gain [in women with a BMI of 18.5–24.9 kg/m^2 (lean)] must include both reduced caloric intake and exercise. This should be the first-line therapy for all women with PCOS for managing long-term consequences.[19]

In terms of weight loss, caloric restriction rather than the composition of the diet is the key factor and smaller trials in women with PCOS have shown no other advantage to a particular hypocaloric diet. Besides caloric restriction, there is no ideal dietary modification in women with PCOS.

Insulin-Sensitizing Agents

Initially the studies focused on insulin sensitizers (agents that improve peripheral insulin sensitivity by lowering circulating insulin levels) including biguanides (metformin) and thiazolidinediones (pioglitazone and rosiglitazone). They rarely cause hypoglycemia, and their individual effects and risk-benefit ratios vary.

At present, data are insufficient to recommend prophylactic insulin-sensitizing agents to prevent diabetes in women with PCOS. There is currently no evidence that the use of insulin-sensitising agents confers any long-term benefit.[19] However, results of diabetes prevention trials may favour more aggressive management when impaired glucose tolerance or metabolic syndrome is present to prevent diabetes.

The drugs which are commonly used to treat PCOS treat the symptoms without targeting the cause. Recently, the drugs which target the root cause, i.e lipotoxicity are used to treat PCOS.

The prime strategy is to reduce the lipid content of non-adipose tissues by either increasing the oxidation of the lipids, or increasing their secretion and transport. Current treatment involves aggressive weight loss.[13]

Another strategy stresses on diverting excess lipids from non-adipose tissues towards the adipose tissues. This is accomplished with thiazolidinediones, a group of medications that activate nuclear receptor proteins responsible for lipid metabolism.[4,13] They are peroxisome proliferator-activated receptor (PPAR) agonists that targets lipotoxicity. By promoting triglycerides storage in adipose tissue, they reduce circulating NEFA thus preventing NEFA exposure in non-adipose tissues.[16]

Rosiglitazone has been found to reduce testosterone levels without affecting insulin levels. Pioglitazone was found to reduce the overexpression of P450c17 induced by MEK/ERK inhibition. There are serious side effects related to these drugs—cardiac complications, bone resorption and even bladder cancer. So, the need to investigate new drug arises to improve lipotoxicity.[16]

Next strategy focuses on inhibiting the apoptotic pathways and signalling cascades which is accomplished by drugs inhibiting the production of specific chemicals required for pathways functioning. Renin–angiotensin system has been implicated in the development of insulin resistance and cardiovascular complications. Angiotensin II mediates its action via angiotensin II type 1 receptors (AT1R) and AT2R. AT1R is expressed in almost all tissues while AT2R is mainly expressed in steroidogenic tissues such as adrenal glands and ovaries. AT1R blockade was shown to improve insulin sensitivity. AT2R inhibits the excessive effects of AT1R activation.[20] A non-peptide drug-like compound, C21/M24, which is a highly selective AT2R agonist has been implicated as a new promising drug. Several animal *in vivo* studies showed that AT2R activation with C21/M24 counteracts many deleterious effects of AT1R activation.[21,22] AT2R stimulation increases PPAR-γ expression and activation. This might be a mechanism by which AT2R improves adipose tissue function.

While this may prove to be the most effective protection against apoptosis, it will require further research and development.

Weight reduction drugs may be useful in reducing hyperandrogenemia. Incretin hormone-based therapies (like exenatide) have been demonstrated to reduce weight and improve insulin resistance in PCOS. However, the clinical experience with these agents in PCOS is limited and significant side-effects may occur; therefore, routine use of incretin based therapies in PCOS is not recommended. Orlistat induces a small weight reduction and improves biochemical hyperandrogenemia but without changing glucose-insulin homeostasis or lipid patterns.[19]

REFERENCES

1. Mc Cartney CR, Marshall JC. Polycystic ovary syndrome. N Engl J Med 2016;375(1):54–64.

2. Roberts CK, Hevener Al, Barnard RJ. Metabolic syndrome and insulin resistance: Underlying causes and modification by exercise training. Compr Physiol.2013;3(1):1–58.

3. Sirmans SM, Pate KA. Epidemiology, diagnosis and management of polycystic ovary syndrome. Clin Epidemiol. 2014;6:1–13.

4. Connally A, Leblanc S, Baillargeon JP. Role of lipotoxicity and contribution of the Renin-Angiotensin system in the development of Polycystic ovary syndrome. Int J Endocrinol. 2018;2018:4315413.

5. Polycystic ovary syndrome. ACOG Practice Bulletin No. 194. Amercian College Of Obstetricians And Gynecologists. 2018;131:e 157–71.

6. Baptiste AG, Battista MC, Trottier A, Baillargeon JP. Insulin and hyperandrogenism in women with polycystic ovary syndrome. J Steroid Biochem Mol Biol. 2010;122:42–52.

7. Nestler JE, Jakubowicz DJ, de Vargas AF, Brik C, Quintero N, Medina F. Insulin stimulates testosterone biosynthesis by human thecal cells from women with polycystic ovary syndrome by activating its own receptor and using inositolglycan mediators as the signal transduction system. J Clin Endocrinol Metab 1998;83:2001–5.

8. Nestler JE, Barlascini CO, Matt DW, Steingold KA, Plymate SR, Clore JN et al. Suppression of serum insulin by diazoxide reduces serum testosterone levels in obese women with polycystic ovary syndrome. JCEM. 1989;68: 1027–32.

9. Kin KN, Rosenfield RN. Role of cytochrome P450c17 in polycystic ovary syndrome. Mol Cell Endocrinol.1998;145:111–21.

10. Penna IA, Canella PR, Reis RM, Silva de Sa MF, Ferriani RA. Acarbose in obese patients with polycystic ovarian syndrome: a double-blind, randomized, placebo-controlled study. Hum Reprod. 2005;20(9):2396–240.

11. Baillargeon JP , Carpentier A. Role of insulin in the hyperandrogenemia of lean women with polycystic ovary syndrome and normal insulin sensitivity. Fertil Steril. 2007;88 (4):886–93.

12. Nestler JE, Powers LP, Matt DW, Steingold KA, Plymate SR, Rittmaster RA et al. A direct effect of hyperinsulinemia on serum sex hormone-binding globulin levels in obese women with the polycystic ovary syndrome. J Clin Endocrinol and Metab. 1991;72:83–9.

13. Available at https: // wikivividly.com/wiki/ Lipotoxicity.

14. Johnson AR, Milner JJ, Makowski L. The inflammation highway: metabolism accelerates inflammatory traffic in obesity. Immunol Rev 2012;249:218–38.

15. Kim JI, Huh JY, Sohn JH, Choe SS, Lee YS, Lim CY, et al. Lipid-overloaded enlarged adipocytes provoke Insulin Resistance independent of inflammation. Mol Cell Biol. 2015;35:1686–99.

16. Faubert J, Battisto MC, Baillargeon JP. Physiology and endocrinology symposium: Insulin action and lipotoxicity in the development of polycystic ovary syndrome: A review. J Anim Sci. 2016;94:1803–11.

17. Bellanger S, Battista MC, Fink GD, Baillargeon JP. Saturated fatty acid exposure induces androgen overproduction in bovine adrenal cells. Steroids. 2012;77:347–53.

18. Alves JPM, Bertolini M, Bertolini LR, Silva CMG, Randina D. Lipotoxicity: Impact on oocyte quality and reproductive efficiency in mammals. Anim Reprod. 2015;12:291–7.

19. Long term consequences of polycystic ovary syndrome. (Greentop guideline No. 33) RCOG. 2014.

20. Jia H, Wang B, Yu L, Jiang Z. Association of angiotensin-converting enzyme gene insertion/deletion polymorphism with polycystic ovary syndrome: a meta-analysis. J Renin-Angiotensin-Aldosterone Sys. 2013;14(3):255–62.

21. Wan Y, Wallinder C, Plouffe B, et al. Design, synthesis, and biological evaluation of the first selective nonpeptide AT2 receptor agonist. J Med Chem. 2004;47(24):5995–6008.

22. Rehman A, Leibowitz A, Yamamoto N, Rautureau Y, Paradis P, Schiffrin EL. Angiotensin type 2 receptor agonist compound 21 reduces vascular injury and myocardial fibrosis in stroke-prone spontaneously hypertensive rats. Hypertension. 2012;59(2):291–9.

7

Role of Vitamin D Deficiency in Pathogenesis of PCOS

Shipra Kunwar

INTRODUCTION

Polycystic ovary syndrome (PCOS) is the most commonly diagnosed female endocrine disorder, with a prevalence rate of nearly 5–10% among women of reproductive age.[1] PCOS is defined by the Rotterdam criteria which includes appearance of at least two of the following criteria:

1. Oligo or ammenorrhoea,
2. Irregular or absent ovulation, and
3. Enlarged ovaries comprising over 12 follicles each.[2]

PCOS is correlated with a variety of cardio-vascular risk factors, such as insulin resistance (IR), impaired glucose tolerance, obesity, hypertension, type 2 diabetes mellitus (T2DM), and metabolic syndrome (MS).[3] IR is the primary metabolic abnormality. IR increases the risk of T2DM and consequently might be the common link between PCOS and T2DM.[4] Insulin resistance leads to hyperinsulinemia which in turn promotes secretion of androgens and also decreases the amount of sex hormone binding globulin (SHBG). All sex hormones such as luteinising hormone, follicle stimulating hormone, estrogen are effected leading to menstrual irregularity and infertility.

Metabolic disturbances and IR in PCOS, might be associated with vitamin D metabolism.

Vitamin D is a steroid hormone synthesised by the body in skin with less than 10–20% coming from diet.[5] The effects of vitamin D are mediated through vitamin D receptor (VDR); which is a member of the steroid/thyroid nuclear hormone receptor superfamily.[6,7] VDR have been identified not only in calcium-regulating tissues such as the intestines, skeleton, and parathyroid glands, but also in many other reproductive organs, such as ovary (particularly granulosa cells), uterus, placenta, testis, hypothalamus, and pituitary.[8–11]

Vitamin D has effects on glucose and insulin metabolism, and low vitamin D status is a risk factor for impaired glucose tolerance, IR and T2DM.[12,13]

Many observational studies suggest a possible deficiency of vitamin D in the causation of PCOS, however, the evidence has been conflicting, a meta-analysis published in 2013 suggested otherwise.[14] A recent meta-analysis showed that 25OH-D concentrations and QUICKI (quantitative insulin sensitivity check index) was lower in subjects with PCOS.[15]

Incidence of vitamin D in general population reported in literature varies from 10–60%.[15,16]

There is a high incidence of obesity in women with PCOS and obesity is an independent risk factor for vitamin D deficiency. Some studies have reported vitamin D levels to 27–56% lower in obese women with PCOs compared to non-obese women with PCOS[17,18] further confirming that obesity is an independent risk factor for vitamin D deficiency. Incidence of vitamin D deficiency in women with PCOS is variously reported as 60–70%[15] with some studies showing no difference in vitamin D levels in women with or without PCOS.

PATHOGENESIS OF PCOS AND ROLE OF VITAMIN D

Vitamin D may play a role in glucose metabolism by enhancing insulin synthesis, release and insulin receptor expression or suppression of proinflammatory cytokines that possibly contribute to the development of insulin resistance.[19]

Vitamin D plays an important role in reproduction, it helps in ovarian follicular development and luteinization via altering anti-Müllerian hormone signaling, follicle stimulating hormone sensitivity and progesterone production in human granulosa cells.[18] This arrest in follicular development is because, vitamin D deficiency leads to increased testosterone levels causing hyperandrogenism.

Advanced glycation end-products (AGEs) have been shown to be involved in the pathogenesis of PCOS, and their serum levels are elevated in women with PCOS.[21] AGEs accumulate in ovarian theca and granulosa layers of women with PCOS.[22]

Another mechanism is reduced vitamin D leads to increased parathormone level which affects glucose metabolism and increases insulin resistance in the body.[23,24]

Vitamin D may stimulate the expression of insulin receptors and thereby enhance insulin responsiveness for glucose transport.[25,26]

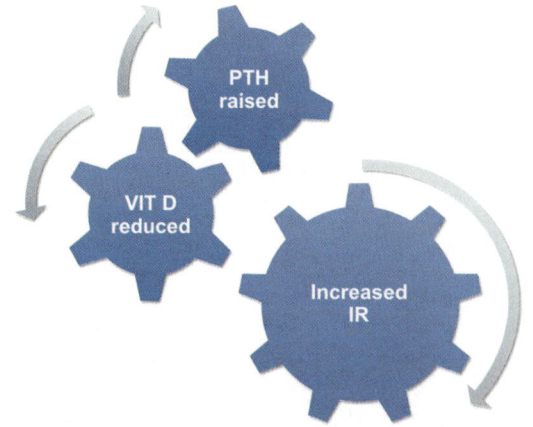

Fig. 7.1: Possible mechanism of reduced IR (insulin resistance)

Vitamin D receptor polymorphism may be related to the pathophysiology of PCOS,[27–29] and VDR-related polymorphism might be involved in PCOS. Multiple VDR susceptibility polymorphisms have been correlated with PCOS parameters, including VDR Apa-I, VDR Cd_2, and VDR Taq-I.

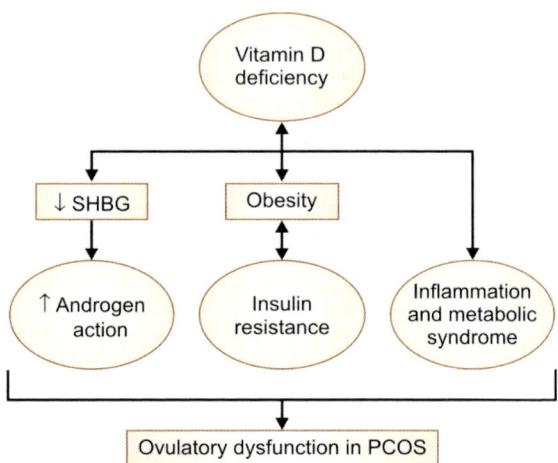

Fig. 7.2: Effects of vitamin D deficiency resulting in PCOS

Association of vitamin D deficiency with factors related to ovulatory dysfunction in polycystic ovary syndrome (PCOS).

Should Women with PCOS be Screened for Vitamin D Levels?

Endocrine Society of North America defined vitamin D deficiency as 25OH-D levels <20 ng/mL and insufficiency as levels of 20–30 ng/mL.[31] Universal screening of vitamin D levels is still not recommended, people at risk of vitamin D deficiency should be screened. As per the endocrine society, screening of vitamin D deficiency is recommended in individuals with rickets, osteomalacia, osteoporosis, chronic kidney disease, hepatic failure, malabsorption syndromes, cystic fibrosis, inflammatory bowel disease, Crohn's disease, bariatric surgery, radiation enteritis, and hyperparathyroidism. Further, it is recommended for

African-American and Hispanic children and adults, pregnant and lactating women, older adults with history of falls, older adults with history of non-traumatic fractures, obese children and adults, and people who are suffering from granuloma.[32]

Screening in PCOS is still not recommended but as obesity is commonly seen in these women it may be helpful investigation.

VITAMIN D SUPPLEMENTATION IN WOMEN WITH PCOS

Vitamin D deficiency has been seen in 20–90%[33] of women in reproductive age group and may be higher upto 100% in India.[34]

Most of vitamin D is synthesized in skin however may not be sufficient and therefore there is requirement of daily supplementation. Institute of medicine (IOM) recommends, adults of age 19 to 70 need a daily supplement of at least 400 IU of vitamin D, and recommended dietary allowance of at least 600 IU.[32,33] Obese adults need at least 2–3 times more vitamin D to treat and prevent vitamin D deficiency.

Though some studies contradict any supplementation with vitamin D helps in PCOS.[15] Irani et al. published an RCT in which vitamin D deficient women with were supplemented with vitamin D for 8 weeks and found substantial improvement in acne, menstrual irregularity, also though none of the women were undergoing infertility treatment 5 women conceived after vitamin D supplementation.[18]

Vitamin D replacement has been shown to have a favourable impact on lipid profile on women with PCOS.[30,35]

For treatment of vitamin D deficiency recommended dose is 4000–6000 IU/day or 60,000 IU weekly for 6 weeks. Though therapeutic supplementation is still under study, a daily dietary supplementation of vitamin D may have a beneficial role.

CONCLUSION

Vitamin D deficiency is rampant especially in Indian subcontinent. Many studies have proven the link between vitamin D deficiency and PCOS beside many other autoimmune and metabolic disorders. So screening women with PCOS for vitamin D deficiency and vitamin D supplementation may go longway in treatment of this chronic disorder, and vitamin D may come out as a relatively safe and cheap medication in PCOS.

REFERENCES

1. Patra SK, Nasrat H, Goswami B, Jain A. Vitamin D as a predictor of insulin resistance polycystic ovarian syndrome. Diabetes Metab Syndr. 2012; 6(3):146–9.

2. The Rotterdam ESHRE/ASRM-Sponsored PCOS consensus workshop group. Revised 2003 consensus on diagnostic criteria and long-term health risks related to polycystic ovary syndrome (PCOS). Hum Reprod. 2004;19(1):41–7.

3. Li HW, Brereton RE, Anderson RA, Wallace AM, Ho CK. Vitamin D deficiency is common and associated with metabolic risk factors in patients with polysyctic ovarian syndrome. Metabolism. 2011; 60(10):1475–81.

4. Ardabili HR, Gargari BP, Farzadi L. Vitamin D supplementation has no effect on insulin resistance assessment in women with polycystic ovary syndrome and vitamin D deficiency. Nutr Res. 2012; 32(3):195–201.

5. Bouillon R, Carmeliet G, Daci E, Segaert S, Verstuyf A. Vitamin D metabolism and action. Osteoporos Int. 1998;8:S13–9.

6. Halloran BP, DeLuca HF. Effect of vitamin D deficiency on fertility and repro-ductive capacity in the female rat. J Nutr 1980;110(8):1573–80.

7. Johnson LE, DeLuca HF. Vitamin D receptor null mutant mice fed high levels of calcium are fertile. J Nutr. 2001;131(6):1787–91.

8. Kinuta K, Tanaka H, Moriwake T, Aya K, Kato S, Seino Y. Vitamin D is an important factor in estrogen biosynthesis of both female and male gonads. Endocrinology. 2000;141(4):1317–24.

9. Hurley WL, Doane RM. Recent developments in the roles of vitamins and minerals in reproduction. J Dairy Sci 1989;72(3):784–804.

10. Halhali A, Acker GM, Garabedian M. 1,25-Dihydroxyvitamin D3 induces in vivo the decidualization of rat endometrial cells. J Reprod Fertil 1991; 91(1):59–64.

11. Harkness LS, Bonny AE. Calcium and vitamin D status in the adolescent: key roles for bone, body weight, glucose tolerance, and estrogen biosynthesis. J Pediatr Adolesc Gynecol 2005; 18(5):305–11.

12. George PS, Pearson ER., Witham MD. Effect of vitamin D supplementation on glycemic control and insulin resistance: a systemic review and meta analysis.Diabet Med 2012; 29(8):142–50.

13. Dalgard C, Petersen MS, Weihe P, Grandjean P. Vitamin D status in relation to glucose metabolism and type 2 diabetes in septuagenarians, Diabetes Care 2011; 34(6):1284–1288.

14. Krul-Poel YH, Sankey C , LouwersY, Lips P, Lambalk CB, Laven JS, et al. The role of vitamin D in metabolic disturbances in polycystic ovary syndrome: a systemic review. Eur J Endocrinol. 2013;169(6):853–65.

15. Xin-Zhuan Jia , Yong-Mei Wang , Na Zhang , Li-Na Guo et al Effect of vitamin D on clinical and biochemical parameters in polycystic ovary syndrome women: A meta analysis. JOGR 2015; 41(11); 1791–1802.

16. Prentice, A. Vitamin D deficiency: a global perspective. Nutrition Reviews (2008) 66, S153–S164.

17. Lips P. Worldwide status of vitamin D nutrition. J Steroid Biochem Mol Biol 2010; 121(1-2):297–300.

18. Irani M and Merhi Z: Role of vitamin D in ovarian physiology and its implication in reproduction: a systematic review. Fertil. Steril., (2014) 102(2):460–468.

19. Hutchinson MS, Grimnes G, Joakimsen RM, Figenschau Y , Jorde R. Low serum 25-hydroxy-vitamin D levels are associated with increased all cause mortality risk in general population: the Tromso study . Eur J Endocrinol 2010; 162(5):935–942.

20. Merhi Z. Advanced glycation end products and their relevance in female reproduction. Hum Reprod 2013; 29(1):135–45.

21. Merhi Z, Irani M, Doswell AD, Ambroggio J. Follicular fluid soluble receptor for glycation end-products (sRAGE): a potential indicator of ovarian reserve. J Clin Endocrinol Metab 2014;99: E 226–33.

22. Diamanti-Kandarakis E, Katsikis I, Piperi C, Kandaraki E, Piouka A, Papavassiliou AG, et al. Increased serum advanced glycation end-products is a distinct finding in lean women with polycystic ovary syndrome (PCOS). Clin Endocrinol (Oxf) 2008;69:634–41.

23. Diamanti-Kandarakis E, Piperi C, Patsouris E, Korkolopoulou P, Panidis D, Pawelczyk L, et al. Immunohistochemical localization of advanced glycation end-products (AGEs) and their receptor (RAGE) in polycystic and normal ovaries. Histochem Cell Biol 2007;127(6): 581–9.

24. Hutchinson MS, Grimnes G, Joakimsen RM, Figenschau Y , Jorde R. Low serum 25-hydroxy-vitamin D levels are associated with increased all cause mortality risk in general population: the Tromso study. Eur J Endocrinol 2010;162(5): 935–942.

25. Tao MF, Zhang Z, Ke YH et al. Association of serum 25-hydroxyvitamin D with the insulin resistance and beta-cell function in a healthy Chinese female population. Acta Pharmacol Sin 2013; 34(8):1070–1074.

26. Maestro B, Campion J, Davila N, Calle C. Stimulation by 1,25-dihydroxyvitamin D3 of insulin receptor expression and insulin responsiveness for glucose transport in U-937 human prototypic cells. Endocr J 2000;47(4):383–91.

27. Maestro B, Davila N, Carranza MC, Calle C. Identification of a Vitamin D response element in the human insulin receptor gene promoter. J Steroid Biochem Mol Biol 2003;84(2-3): 223–30.

28. Hahn S, Haselhorst U, Tan S, Quadbeck B, Schmidt M, Roesler S, et al. Low serum 25-hydroxyvitamin D concentrations are associated with insulin resistance and obesity in women with polycystic ovary syndrome. Exp Clin Endocrinol Diabetes 2006;114(10):577–83.

29. Mahmoudi T. Genetic variation in the vitamin D receptor and polycystic ovary syndrome risk. Fertil Steril 2009;92(4):1381–3.

30. Ranjzad F, Mahban A, Shemirani AI, Mahmoudi T, Vahedi M, Nikzamir A, et al. Influence of gene variants related to calcium homeostasis on biochemical parameters of women with polycystic ovary syndrome. J Assist Reprod Genet 2011; 28(3):225–32.

31. Holick MF, Binkley NC, Bischoff-Ferrari HA, Gordon CM, Hanley DA, Heaney RP, et al. Evaluation, treatment, and prevention of vitamin D deficiency: an Endocrine Society clinical practice guideline. J Clin Endocrinol Metab 2011; 96(7):1911–30.

32. Holick MF, Binkley NC, Bischoff-Ferrari HA, et al. Evaluation, treatment, and prevention of vitamin D deficiency: An Endocrine Society clinical practice guideline. J Clin Endocrin Metab 2011; 96(7):1911–30.

33. Balasubramanian S, Dhanalakshmi K, Amperayani S. Vitamin D deficiency in childhood—A review of current guidelines on diagnosis and management. *Indian Pediatr* 2013; 50(7):669–75.

34. Vitamin D Deficiency in India: Prevalence, Causalities and Interventions Nutrients. 2014 Feb; 6(2): 729–775. Published online 2014 Feb 21. doi: 10.3390/nu6020729.

35. Nasri K, Akrami S, Rahimi M, Taghizadeh M, Behfar M, Mazandaranian MR et al–The effects of vitamin D and primose oil co-supplementation on lipid profiles and biomarkers of oxidative stress in vitamin D-deficient women with PCOS:A Randomised, double-blind, placebo-controlled trial. Endorcr Res 2018;43(1):1–10.

Metabolic Consequences of PCOS

Hiralal Konar, Picklu Chaudhuri, Arindam Halder

OVERVIEW

Our first knowledge about polycystic ovarian syndrome came from a case series report by Dr Irving F Stein and Dr Michael Leventhal in 1935. They demonstrated a triad of polycystic ovaries, hirsutism and oligo-/amenorrhea in a series of women and successfully treated them by wedge resection of ovary thus giving an idea that the disease is ovarian in origin.[1] After that, the subject received tremendous attention by researchers all over the globe and about 28,000 research articles were published on this topic in subsequent 80 years, majority of them in the last 15 years. Thanks to all these researches, the perception regarding the pathophysiology of the disease has changed and it is now considered a multisystem, metabolic and endocrine disease with reproductive implications.

INCIDENCE

The prevalence of PCOS according to diagnostic criteria of NIH, Rotterdam and AE-PCOS society were 6%, 10% and 10%, respectively as described in a meta-analysis.[2] Indian studies reported a higher prevalence ranging from 2.2 to 26%.[3] So, about 1 in 5–17 women is suffering from this condition. The high prevalence may be due to unhealthy lifestyle including fast food, lack of exercise and sedentary habits. It may also be due to increased awareness and improved accessibility to medical care.

METABOLIC SYNDROME AND PCOS

There are different criteria for diagnosis of metabolic syndrome (Table 8.1).

The metabolic syndrome, although varies in diagnostic criteria, has 4 major components—

TABLE 8.1: Definitions of metabolic syndrome for women, according to WHO, NCEP ATP III and IDF criteria

WHO	NCEP ATP III	IDF
IFG or IGT of insulin resistance plus ≥2 of the following: • BMI >30 kg/m² or WHR >0.85 • HDL <1.0 mmol/L (<40 mg/dL) • TG ≥1.7 mmol/L (150 mg/dL) • BP ≥140/90 mm Hg or use of blood pressure medication • Microalbuminuria >20 pg/min • Alb/crea ratio ≥30 mg/g	≥3 of following: • WC ≥88 cm • HDL <1.3 mmol/L (<50 mg/dL) • TG ≥1.7 mmoVL (150 mg/dL) • BP ≥135/85 mmHg or use of blood pressure medication	Central obesity defined as WC above the ethnicity specific cut-off plus ≥2 of the following: • TG ≥1.7 mmol/L (150 mg/dL) or specific treatment • HDL <1.3 mmol/L (<50 mg/dL) or specific treatment • BP ≥135/85 mm Hg or use of blood pressure medication • Fasting plasma glucose ≥5.6 mmol/L (100 mg/dL) or previously diagnosed T2D

BP = blood pressue; HDI = high density lipoprotein cholesterol; IGT = impaired glucose tolerance; T2D = type 2 diabetes; TG = triglycerine; WC = waist circumference; WHR = waist to hip ratio, WHO = World Health Organization; NCEP ATP III = National Cholesterol Education Programme Adult Treatment Panel III; IDF = International Diabetic Federation) obesity, insulin resistance/impaired glucose tolerance/type 2 diabetes mellitus, dyslipidemia, and hypertension. PCOS is intimately related to all these components as follows.

PCOS AND OBESITY

35–60% women with PCOS are obese and 28% of all obese women have PCOS. Obesity is the cause and not the effect of PCOS. There are 3 distinct mechanisms by which obesity is involved in the pathogenesis of PCOS—first, by increasing aromatization of androgen to estrogen in the adipose tissue leading to hyperestrogenism and chronic anovulation; second, by decreasing sex hormone-binding globulin (SHBG) thus increasing the free estrogen and androgen level and third, by causing impaired glucose tolerance leading to hyperinsulinemia which causes increased androgen production in the ovary.

Hence, a weight reduction even to the extent of 2–5% is beneficial in restoring ovulation and regularizing menstrual cycle and improving metabolic consequences.

Insulin Resistance/Impaired Glucose Tolerance/Type 2 Diabetes Mellitus and PCOS

Fifty to seventy-five percent of women with PCOS have insulin resistance, 35% have IGT and 10% have DM

Prevalence of PCOS is sixfold higher in women with type 2 DM.

Insulin resistance leads to compensatory hyperinsulinemia which acts on the ovary through IGF-1 receptors resulting increased androgen production in the ovary. Apart from that, insulin causes decreased production of SHBG from liver and thus increasing free androgen and oestrogen level. This hyperandrogenemia in turn aggravates insulin resistance further. So, this becomes a vicious cycle.

Dyslipidemia and PCOS

Seventy percent of PCOS cases have at least one abnormal lipid parameter[4] and it may be due to insulin resistance, increased androgen and increased oestrogen.

Hypertension and PCOS

Hypertension is 3 times more common in PCOS. Although there is no direct evidence of increased incidence of cardiovascular disease, dyslipidemia increases the risk of premature atherosclerosis in PCOS.

Apart from these, PCOS is related to the following multisystem dysfunction.

Liver Disease

Non-alcoholic fatty liver disease (NAFLD)/ alcoholic steatohepatitis (NASH): Incidence of NAFLD is 15–57.8% (based on elevated transaminases) and 60–70% (on USG) among obese PCOS and 39% among lean PCOS.[5]

Dermatological Problems

PCOS is associated with acne in 67.5%, hirsutism in 62.5%, seborrhea in 52.5%, alopecia in 30% and acanthosis nigricans in 22.5% cases.[6]

Psychosexual Problems

Depression, anxiety, eating disorders, sexual problems, low self-esteem are common but undiagnosed entities associated with PCOS leading to reduced quality of life (QoL).[7]

Obstructive Sleep Apnea (OSA)

Although the incidence is high in obese PCOS, it remains often undiagnosed. OSA is a risk factor for HT, stroke, CV disease, and pulmonary HT.

PCOS and Cancer

Risk of endometrial cancer is increased by 2.89-fold in women with PCOS due to effect of unopposed estrogen and risk increases in women with less than 4 periods/year.[8] However, there is no additional risk for breast and ovarian cancers.

MANAGEMENT GUIDELINES[9]

Although, women with PCOS come to the gynecologist for menstrual and infertility-related problems, but the duty of the gynecologist is beyond regularization of her menstrual cycle and inducing her ovulation. They should screen for metabolic and multi-system diseases, counsel and make them aware regarding the long term health hazards. Treat and refer to the concerned specialists as required.

Screen

It is necessary to clinically assess obesity by BMI and waist-hip ratio and hypertension by regular BP measurement.

USG upper abdomen and liver function tests, oral glucose tolerance test, and lipid profile are very important screening tests.

TVS for endometrial thickness and endometrial sampling is necessary in older women with PCOS who have infrequent periods in order to rule out endometrial hyperplasia and cancer.

Counsel

One need to elicit history of OSA (sleep disturbance, fatigue, snoring) and psychological problems (depression, lack of interest, etc). It is very important to make the women aware regarding long-term health hazards of PCOS.

Treat

First line of therapy is lifestyle modification, by diet control and exercise. Low calorie diet and avoidance of fast food is necessary. Brisk walking for at least 30 min/day is to be advised.

Refer

A multidisciplinary approach in managing metabolic and multisystem disorders with metabolic specialist and endocrinologist, gastroenterologist, pulmonologist, nutritionist and psychiatrist may be required according to individual need.

REFERENCES

1. Amenorrhea associated with bilateral polycystic ovaries lF. Stein M.D. MichaelL. Leventhal M.D. Am J of Obst and Gynecol. Volume 29, Issue 2, 1935, Pages 181–91.
2. The prevalence and phenotypic features of polycystic ovary syndrome: a systematic review and meta-analysis. Bozdag G, Mumusoglu S, Zengin D, Karabulut E, Yildiz BO. Hum Reprod. 2016 Dec;31(12):2841–55. Epub 2016 Sep 22.
3. Prevalence of polycystic ovarian syndrome in Indian adolescents. Nidhi R, Padmalatha V, Nagarathna R, Amritanshu R. J PediatrAdolesc Gynecol. 2011 Aug;24(4):223–7. doi: 10.1016/j.JPAG.2011.03.002. Epub 2011 May 19.
4. Prevalence and predictors of dyslipidemia in women with polycystic ovary syndrome. RS Legro, AR Kunselman, ADunaif . Am J of Med 2001;111:607–13.
5. Nonalcoholic fatty liver disease and polycystic ovary syndrome. Evangeline Vassilatou; World J of Gastroenterology. 2014 Jul 14; 20(26): 8351–63.
6. Correlation of Skin Changes with Hormonal Changes in Polycystic Ovarian Syndrome: A Cross-sectional Study Clinical Study. Gowri BV, Chandravathi PL, Sindhu PS, Naidu KS.Indian J Dermatol. 2015 Jul-Aug;60(4):419. doi: 10.4103/0019-5154.160505.
7. Polycystic ovary syndrome and mental health: A review. Himelein MJ, Thatcher SS. Obstet Gynecol Surv. 2006 Nov;61(11):723–32.
8. Evaluating the association between endometrial cancer and polycystic ovary syndrome. Haoula Z, Salman M, Atiomo W. Hum Reprod. 2012 May;27(5):1327–31. doi: 10.1093/humrep/des042. Epub 2012 Feb 24.
9. Polycystic Ovary Syndrome, Long-term Consequences (Green-top Guideline No. 33).

Infertility and Adverse Pregnancy Outcomes in PCOS

Richa Kansal

Polycystic ovarian syndrome (PCOS), a heterogenous condition characterizied by hyperandrogenism, ovarian dysfunction and polycystic ovarian morphology, is one of the most common endocrinopathy affecting females of reproductive life (incidence ranging from 5–13%),[1,2] with effects extending not only to this era but also to the post-reproductive life (Dunaif and Fauser, 2013; Orio and Palomba, 2014).[3,4] The disorder has been implicated with ovulatory dysfunction, infertility, hirsutism, and lately with early and late adverse pregnancy outcome along with long-term compilations like diabetes mellitus, cardiac manifestation, and metabolic syndrome.

The direct effect of PCOS is most evident on the reproductive performance of the lady. The clinical presentation usually includes: Menstrual irregularities, usually oligomenorrhea, or amenorrhea associated with clinical or/and biochemical evidences of hyperandorgenesis. The individual may be obese (50–70%) with increased BMI. Hyperinsulinemia/insulin resistance (IR), present both in obese (80%) and non-obese (30–40%) women with PCOS, is more strongly associated with anovulation. IR plays role in obesity, increased BMI and high circulating levels of plasminogen activator inhibitor-1 in the body, all of which can result in early pregnancy loss. Abnormal gonadotropin secretion, hyperandrogenism and metabolic abnormalities along with genetic,[5] environmental, clinical, and other biochemical factors involved in this complex

condition lead to infertility commonly seen in these individuals along with possible pregnancy complications and long-term health problems in both mother and child.

INFERTILITY IN PCOS

In addition to menstrual irregularities, Infertility forms the commonest presentation with which the females affected with PCOS seek medical attention.[6] Although a subset of these females may achieve pregnancy without any intervention (Hudecova, et al. 2009), majority have anovulation which forms the commonest cause of infertility in women with PCOS (Teede, et al. 2010). Altered gonadotropin secretion, ovarian hyperandrogenism and hyperinsulinemia may promote premature granulosa cell luteinization and affect oocyte quality. The intrafollicular environment is further affected by the paracrine dysregulation of growth factors, which may also result in impaired cytoplasmic and/or nuclear maturation of oocytes (Dumesic, et al. 2008). Endometrial receptivity is also seen to be altered in these patients with endometrial dysfunction resulting in a variety of changes in endometrial histomorphology and receptivity markers. Obesity and IR both adversely affect reproductive performance of the lady. Lately studied, the genetic aspect of the disease etiology further adds to the complexity of the situation.

As has already been discussed in great detail in previous chapters, the syndrome with its hetrogenous etiology and variability in phenotype expression and altered expression of genes affecting signal transduction pathways continues to challenge complete understanding of the disease so as to render the treatment more empirical.

PCOS is the commonest cause of anovulatory infertility but as discussed earlier available evidences suggest that other factors also add to subfertility in these patients. The treatment is mainly directed towards achieving ovulation in these patients. Correcting the obesity, metabolic and endocrine abnormalities also help in achieving pregnancy.

Confirming the diagnosis of PCOS is the first challenge. Women may first learn about being affected by PCOS when they present to gynecology clinic with infertility. The workup includes (Australian NHMRC, the ESHRE, and the ASRE, 2018):

- Detailed history (including menstrual irregularities, obstetric performance, metabolic disorders, family history). Anxiety and depressive symptoms should be screened.
- Confirming the diagnosis of PCOS using Rotterdam's criteria (presence of 2 out of 3 criteria):
  1. Oligo- and/or anovulation
  2. Clinical or biochemical hyperandrogenism
  3. Polycystic ovaries (≥12 follicles measuring 2–9 mm and/or ovarian volume ≥10 mL)
- Weight, height, waist circumference, BMI.
- Transvaginal ultrasound to identify multicystic ovaries and to document anovulation, if present.
- Serum FSH and LH levels, TSH.
- Free testosterone levels, free androgen index.
- Androstenedione and dehydroepiandrosterone sulfate (DHEAS) levels—other causes of hyperandrogenism need to be ruled out.
- Glycemic status.

- Lipid profile in overweight and obese women with PCOS.
- Investigations to rule out other causes of infertility.

The evaluation of infertility in women with PCOS or other causes of subfertility should start after six months of attempting pregnancy without success, if the couple has regular sexual intercourse (2 to 3 times/week) without using contraceptive methods (ASRM, 2013). Efficacy of the treatment of infertile women with PCOS requires optimization by evaluations of tubal patency (hysterosalpingography or laparoscopy with chromotubation) and semen analysis (spermogram), and hence these investigations are mandatory before deciding on treatment.

Treatment initially includes preconception guidelines, such as lifestyle changes (weight loss/physical exercise), folic acid therapy to prevent the risk of fetal neural tube defects and halting the consumption of tobacco and alcohol.[7]

- *Weight loss:* The gold standard for improving insulin sensitivity in obese PCOS should be weight loss, by diet and exercise. Weight loss (even 5 to 10% of body weight) itself can improve the endocrinal aspects in PCOS and result in lowering the androgen levels with spontaneous resumption of menses (Vause, et al. 2009).[8]

Clomiphene citrate along with timed intercourse is the first-line pharmacological treatment for inducing ovulation. The second-line pharmacological treatment includes the administration of exogenous gonadotropins or laparoscopic ovarian surgery (ovarian drilling, LOD).[9]

- Ovulation induction with timed intercourse forms the mainstay of treatment. Clomiphene citrate (CC) is the preferred choice to achieve ovulation when anovulation is the sole cause of infertility.[10,11] As per Australian NHMRC, the ESHRE, and the ASRE guidelines, 2018, letrozole should be considered the first-line pharmacologic agent for ovulation induction in women with PCOS.

- Gonadotropins form the second line of ovulation induction therapy, if CC/letrozole fails to achieve ovulation induction in these cases. The possibility of multiple pregnancy and ovarian hyperstimulation syndrome is high particularly in women with PCOS while using these agents and for these caution is warranted.

- *Insulin sensitizers:* Treatment with metformin, a biguanide agent that enhances the action of insulin at the cellular level, may improve the hyperinsulinemia and hyperandrogenemia with improvement in the menstrual abnormalities and subsequent conception in women with PCOS.[9] When metformin is used alone as an ovulation induction agent, ovulation rates are typically between 30 and 40%, but evidence for a significant increase in pregnancy rates is lacking. The success rate approaches 90% with CC.

- Corticosteroids can be added only in cases where there is an increased DHEAS levels, as this will suggest an increase in the adrenal androgens which is sometimes seen in patients of PCOS. The most widely used protocol includes dexamethasone administered at night-time in a dose of 0.5 mg orally in conjunction with clomiphene citrate treatment.

- *Laparoscopic ovarian surgery (ovarian drilling):* First described in 1939 via wedge resection has now been replaced with ovarian drilling (max. 5 in an ovary) in cases not responding to medications (SOGC, laparoscopic ovarian drilling may be considered in women with clomiphene-resistant PCOS, especially in the presence of other laparoscopic indications). Destruction of androgen producing theca cells and normalized ovarian milieu may be responsible for successful ovulation seen after the procedure. A small French study[12] also suggested that surgical management via ovarian drilling with hydrolaparoscopy

may be beneficial in cases of PCOS that are resistant to clomiphene citrate. Multiple pregnancy rates are lower with ovarian drilling than with gonadotropin treatment (1% vs 16%, respectively), but there are ongoing concerns about potential complications which include formation of adhesions and ovarian atrophy and concerns regarding the long-term effects of ovarian drilling on ovarian function.[13]

The common technique of LOD is the use of monopolar electrocautery (diathermy) or laser with comparable results. Normally, three to eight diathermy punctures are performed in each ovary using 600–800 J energy for each puncture, lead to further normal ovulation in 74% of the cases in the next 3–6 months. More than eight punctures seem to increase the occurrence of postoperative pelvic adhesions and decrease the ovarian reserve.[14–16]

- *In vitro* fertilization (IVF) is reserved for women with PCOS and unsuccessful gonadotropin therapy or those with other indications for this procedure.[17] Chen et al studied frozen-embryo transfer among infertile women with PCOS. The frozen-embryo transfers were associated with a higher rate of live birth, a lower risk of the ovarian hyperstimulation syndrome, but a higher risk of pre-eclampsia after the first transfer than was fresh-embryo transfer.

- Treatment of other metabolic or endocrine abnormalities is also required, if found associated like hyperandrogenemia, impaired glucose tolerance—while planning for pregnancy.

Follow-up with USG to document the growing follicle and treatment as per the clinical presentation/and other factors of infertility present.

Live birth is achieved within 2 years in about 80% of women with PCOS undergoing treatment (Veltman-Verhulst et al, 2012).

The risk for gestational diabetes, preeclampsia, cesarean delivery, and preterm and post-term delivery is higher in pregnancies of PCOS women. In addition, their newborns are at increased risk of being large for gestational age, but they are not at increased risk of stillbirth or neonatal death.[18]

PREGNANCY COMPLICATION IN PATIENTS WITH PCOS

Majority of studies on PCOS have focused on diagnosis, menstrual irregularities, hirsutism and infertility with little attention to pregnancy complications and subsequent child outcomes. Intriguingly, complications do not seem to stop once a woman with PCOS conceives, since she will be at a higher risk of miscarriage, both after spontaneous or assisted conception (ART) and a closer pregnancy follow-up should be provided to these patients. (Amsterdam ESHRE/ASRM-Sponsored 3rd PCOS consensus Workshop Group, 2012). Four systemic reviews with meta-analyses (Boomsma et al., 2006; Kjerul et al., 2011; Qin et al., 2013, Hai-Feng, et al. 2016) all calculated increased risk of pregnancy-induced hypertension (3.07–4.07 OR), pre-eclampsia (3.28–4.23 OR), gestational diabetes (2.81–2.94 OR) and premature delivery (1.34–2.20 OR) in women with PCOS. But in these studies data had not been adjusted for BMI, and other confounding factors.[19,20]

Adverse pregnancy outcomes like multiple pregnancy, early pregnancy loss (EPL), pregnancy-induced hypertension (PIH) and pre-eclampsia (PE), gestational diabetes mellitus (GDM), preterm delivery, cesarean delivery and probable adverse fetal outcomes and perinatal death have all gained attention in the recent years with probable association in pregnancy with PCOS documented (Hai-Feng, et al. 2016). Characteristic features of PCOS, such as hyperandrogenism, obesity, insulin resistance and metabolic abnormalities, may contribute to this increased risk of obstetric and neonatal complications.[19] Complications inherent to conception after infertility management (Pinborg et al, 2013;

Malchau et al, 2014), potential higher rate of multiple pregnancy (Johnston et al, 2014) and factors like time-to-pregnancy (Messerlian et al, 2013), also play a role in these patients and warrant due attention while interpreting data available.

Etiology

1. *Obesity:* BMI >25 has significantly higher odds of miscarriage regardless of method of conception (Metwally, et al. 2008), PIH and PE (Sween, et al. 2015), assisted vaginal delivery and cesarean delivery (Dietz, et al. 2005; Yu, et al. 2006), GDM (Yogev and Catalano, 2009) and other adverse effects on pregnancy and fetus. A weight loss of 10 kg with a 6-month lifestyle intervention resulted in significant reduction of pregnancy complications including early pregnancy losses (Clark, et al. 1998).

2. *Hyperinsulinemia:* Insulin Resistance forms an independent risk factor for adverse pregnancy outcomes (Tian, et al. 2007). Its association with obesity and high circulating levels of plasminogen activator-1 (Glueck, et al. 1999) which in themselves add to the risk (Wang, et al. 2002). IR independently increases eightfold the risk of spontaneous abortion after ART, suggestion to be one of the main risk factors for EPL. A fact supported by the findings of a meta-analysis including 1106 patients with PCOS which calculated that the risk of EPL could be reduced by about 70% when using metformin.

3. *LH hypersecretion:* Elevated LH levels in early follicular phase have been shown to be associated with increased EPL in both natural (Regan, et al. 1990) and ovulation induction cycles (Homburg et al, 1988; Hamilton-Fairley, et al. 1992). A fact supported by the effect of laparoscopic ovarian drilling, which has been shown to reduce EPL by lowering LH secretion (Ar and Lachelin, 1993).

4. *Hyperandrogenism:* Levels are increased throughout pregnancy (Falbo, et al. 2010)

with postulated abnormal steroidogenic function (Escobar, et al. 2011) of the placenta in women with PCOS (Malinqueo, et al. 2013). Altered early trophoblast invasion and placentation (Palomba, et al. 2012d, 2013a, 2014c) due to direct effect of androgens on the endometrium and/or to a specific tissue susceptibility (Cakmak and Taylor, 2011; Kajihara, et al. 2013), impairment of nutrient transport across placenta (Falbo, et al. 2010), sympathetic and vascular hyperactivity (Shobel, et al. 1996), altered metabolism (Berger, et al. 1984; Sir-Petermann, et al. 2005), and effect on cervical remodeling and myometrial function (Makieva et al, 2014) are the possible mechanisms by which hyperandrogenism with PCOS influences pregnancy outcome.

5. *Plasminogen activator-1 (PAI-1):* Elevated levels are associated with increased rate of EPL and various obstetric complications (Glueck, et al. 1999).

6. *Endometrial dysfunction:* Impaired endometrial receptivity and reduced endometrial blood flow occur most probably due to hyperinsulinemia and insulin resistance, decreased glycodelin and insulin-like growth factor binding protein-1 (IGFBP-1) (Jakubowicz et al, 2001) and increased endothelin-1 (ET-1) (Diamantis-Kandarakis, et al. 2005).

7. *Placental changes:* Histopathological examination shows chronic changes in villi suggestive of local microvascular and inflammatory damage (Palomba, et al. 2013a).

ADVERSE PREGNANCY OUTCOMES

Early Pregnancy Loss

There are two Australian studies available in literature demonstrating that early pregnancy loss is more prevalent among women with PCOS (admission rate for miscarriages 11.1% for PCOS vs 6.1% for controls, Hart et al, 2015; miscarriage rates 20% for PCOS vs 14.9% for controls, Joham, et al. 2014). Interestingly, isolated PCOS was not related with increased

miscarriage rate because when use of fertility treatment was included in the model (ovulation induction and/or IVF), the association fall short. Fertility treatment and BMI in the overweight and obese groups have been found to be independently associated with pregnancy loss, multiple pregnancy and to the loads of other pregnancy related problems suggesting an indirect association, effect of phenotype, or other factors yet poorly understood. In PCOS women, though exact mechanism remains unclear, IR and hyperandrogenemia have also been linked to increased risk of recurrent pregnancy loss (RPL, loss of 3 or more consecutive pregnancies) (prevalence of RPL in infertile patients 40% PCOS group vs 12 % non-PCOS group, Banu, et al. 2014) with increased prevalence of IR as compared to controls (Craig, et al. 2002) and possible prognostic value of elevated free androgen index for subsequent miscarriage in these women (Cocksedge, et al. 2008).

Multiple Pregnancy

Ovulation induction protocols for anovulatory infertility in women with PCOS are commonly associated with multiple pregnancy, which in turn forms an important cause of increased adverse pregnancy outcomes like small for gestational age infants (10-fold increased risk), premature delivery (6-fold) (Rao, et al. 2001; Society of Obstetricians and Gynaecologists of Canada, 2014), and perinatal mortality (Rao, et al. 2004). Risks of preterm and low birth weight infants delivered to women with history of PCOS, after adjusting for BMI and gestational age, were not statistically significant (Løvvik, et al. 2015).

Pregnancy-Induced Hypertension and Pre-Eclampsia

Significant risk of PIH (12.7% vs 5.3%) and PE (8% vs 2%) has been associated with PCOS (Palomba et al, 2014a,b). Data collected on other studies though showing a significant association with PIH. Hai-Feng, et al. (2016) in a meta-analysis have concluded a higher risk (PE: RR:2.79; 95%CI: 2.29-3.38; p<0.001, PIH: RR: 2.46; 95% CI: 1.95-3.09; p<0.001).

Gestational Diabetes Mellitus

It is the most commonly described pregnancy complication in women with PCOS and has substantial data to support a higher risk after adjusting for age, BMI, hypertension, smoking and demographic factors (2 times higher OR 2.32, 95% CI 1.88–2.88, Roos, et al. 2011; OR 2.1, 95% CI 1.1–3.9, Joham, et al. 2014b) implicating PCOS as an independent risk factor. A recent meta-analysis (Hai-Feng, et al. 2016) has demonstrated increased risk of GDM (RR: 2.78; 95% CI: 2.27–3.40; P < 0.001). Suspecting the condition is important in improving the prognosis of both mother and baby as an early diagnosis and careful management significantly reduces complications in both (Ngai et al, 2014; Poolsup, et al. 2014).

Other Maternal Complications

Increased risk of delivery by cesarean section: Data is controversial. PCOS in pregnancy might affect the incidence of cesarean delivery (RR: 1.25; 95% CI: 1.15–1.36; p <0.001, Hai-Feng, et al. 2016). Boomsma et al, 2006 have reported a significantly higher risk of delivery by cesarean section in women with PCOS while other meta-analyses fail to demonstrate so (Kjerulff, et al. 2011; Qin, et al. 2013).

Fetal Complications

Pregnancy in PCOS women has been found to have an increased risk of hypoglycemia (RR: 2.85; 95% CI: 1.93–4.22; p<0.001) and perinatal death (RR: 1.83; 95% CI: 1.06–3.16; p = 0.029) (Hai-Feng et al, 2016). Other available data show an increased frequency of preterm delivery (OR 2.21, 95% CI, 1.69–2.90, Roos et al, 2011; OR 2.28, 95% CI, 1.51–3.45, Naver et al, 2014) with the risk confined to androgenic women with PCOS (OR 2.78 vs 1.35 for non-androgenic women), and meconium aspiration (OR 2.02, 95% CI, 1.33–3.61, Roos, et al. 2011). The data regarding small for gestational age infant is conflicting.

Hai-Feng, et al. (2016) in a meta-analysis demonstrated no or little effect of PCOS on other parameters studied such as oligohydramnios, polyhydramnios, large for gestational age infants, small for gestational age infants, fetal growth restriction, preterm premature membrane rupture, fasting blood glucose, high-density lipoprotein, low-density lipoprotein, triglyceride, total cholesterol, congenital malformation, macrosomia and respiratory distress syndrome but accepted availability of limited data, small studies, effect weakened by potential confounders, and inter-relationship of various factors, e.g. BMI levels, glucose metabolic impairment, GDM, adverse maternal and fetal outcomes; infertility treatment protocols and multiple pregnancy and its inherent risks, as the limitation of their study.

Prevention and Management

1. Preconception weight loss (Agha, et al. 2014)
2. *Avoid excess weight gain during pregnancy:* Dietary modification and/or physical activity intervention (Agha, et al. 2014)
3. Screening for pre-gestational diabetes (Peterson, et al. 2015)
4. Avoidance of multiple pregnancy particularly in infertility treated patients (Løvvik, et al. 2015)
5. Early detection and prompt treatment of pregnancy complications
6. Metformin is effective and safe for the treatment of GDM (Balsells, et al. 2015), particularly in overweight and obese. As far its role with prevention of pregnancy complications is concerned, benefit is not conclusive.

CONCLUSION

Polycystic ovarian syndrome is a significant public health problem having reproductive, metabolic and psychological implications. Its hetrogenous etiology and diverse presentation presents a clinical challenge across the life course which is exacerbated by a lack of complete understanding of its affection. PCOS has long been recognised as an important cause of infertility. Now there is sufficient evidence to suggest its role in adverse pregnancy outcomes. There is a compelling need to identify the gaps in knowledge and intensify the efforts to better understand the disease as the list of affections due to PCOS is ever growing and providing best practice and evidence based care is our responsibility.

REFERENCES

1. Revised 2003 consensus on diagnostic criteria and long-term health risks related to polycystic ovary syndrome (PCOS). Rotterdam ESHRE/ASRM-Sponsored PCOS consensus workshop group. Hum Reprod 2004;19(1):41–7.

2. Melo AS, Vieira CS, Barbieri MA, Rosa-E-Silva AC, Silva AA, Cardoso VC, Reis RM, Ferriani RA, Silva-de-Sá MF, Bettiol H. High prevalence of polycystic ovary syndrome in women born small for gestational age. Hum Reprod 2010; 25(8): 2124–31.

3. Dunaif A, and Fauser BCJM. Renaming PCOS– A two-state solution. Journal of Clinical Endocrinology and Metabolism 2013;98(11): 4325–4328.

4. Orio F, Palomba S. Reproductive endocrinology: New guidelines for the diagnosis and treatment of PCOS. Nat Rev Endocrinol. 2014; 10(3):130–32.

5. Ehrmann DA, Kasza K, Azziz R, Legro RS, Ghazzi MN. Effects of race and family history of type 2 diabetes on metabolic status of women with polycystic ovary syndrome. J Clin Endocrinol Metab 2005; 90(1):66–71.

6. Azziz R, Woods KS, Reyna R, Key TJ, Knochenhauer ES, Yildiz BO. The prevalence and features of the polycystic ovary syndrome in an unselected population. J Clin Endocrinol Metab. 2004; 89(6):2745–49.

7. Anderson Sanches Melo, Rui Alberto Ferriani, Paula Andrea Navarro. Treatment of infertility in women with polycystic ovary syndrome: approach to clinical practice. Clinics (Sao Paulo). 2015; 70(11): 765–769.

8. Vause TD, Cheung AP, Sierra S, et al. Ovulation induction in polycystic ovary syndrome. J Obstet Gynaecol Can 2010; 32(5):495–502.

9. American College of Obstetricians and Gynecologists. Polycystic ovary syndrome. Washington, DC: American College of Obstetricians and Gynecologists; 2009. ACOG practice bulletin; no. 108.

10. Thessaloniki ESHRE/ASRM- Sponsored PCOS Consensus Workshop Group (2008) Consensus on infertility treatment related to Polycystic Ovary Syndrome. Hum Reprod 2013; 23(3):462–77.

11. Perales-Puchalt A, Legro RS. Ovulation induction in women with polycystic ovary syndrome. Steroids. 2013;78(8):767–72.

12. Poujade O, Gervaise A, Faivre E, Deffieux X, Fernandez H. Surgical management of infertility due to polycystic ovarian syndrome after failure of medical management. Eur J Obstet Gynecol Reprod Biol 2011; 158(2):242–47.

13. Farquhar C, Brown J, Marjoribanks J. Laparoscopic drilling by diathermy or laser for ovulation induction in anovulatory polycystic ovary syndrome. Cochrane Database Syst Rev. 2014;6:CD001122.

14. Aakvaag A, Gjonnaess H. Hormonal response to electrocautery of the ovary in patients with polycystic ovarian disease. Br J Obstet Gynaecol 1985; 92(12):1258–64.

15. Unlu C, Atabekoglu CS. Surgical treatment in polycystic ovary syndrome. Curr Opin Obstet Gynecol 2006; 18(3):286–92.

16. Al-Inany HG, Youssef MA, Aboulghar M, Broekmans F, Sterrenburg M, Smit J, et al. Gonadotrophin-releasing hormone antagonists for assisted reproductive technology. Cochrane Database Syst Rev. 2011; 5:CD001750.

17. Roos N, Kieler H, Sahlin L, et al. Risk of adverse pregnancy outcomes in women with polycystic ovary syndrome: population based cohort study. BMJ 2011; 343:d6309.

18. Stefano Palomba , Marlieke A de Wilde, Angela Falbo, Maria PH Koster, Giovanni Battista La Sala, Bart CJM Fauser. Pregnancy complications in women with polycystic ovary syndrome. Human Reproduction Update 2015; 21(5):575–592.

19. Grewal, PerbinderYu, Hai-Feng MS; Chen, Hong-Su MS; Rao, Da-Pang MS; Gong, Jian MS. Association between polycystic ovary syndrome and the risk of pregnancy complications: A PRISMA-compliant systematic review and meta-analysis. Medicine 2016; 95(51):e4863.

20. Apostolos Tsironis. "Polycystic Ovary Syndrome and Early Pregnancy Loss: A Review Article". EC Gynaecology 7.2 (2018):35–42.

PCOS: Symptomatology, Types and Diagnosis

Jai Bhagwan Sharma, Monica Gupta

INTRODUCTION

Polycystic ovarian syndrome (PCOS) is the most common endocrine disorder affecting 5–10% women of reproductive age.[1] It was first described by Stein and Leventhal in 1935 as a syndrome complex which included enlarged ovaries, oligomenorrhea or amenorrhea and hirsutism.[2] Ovarian wedge resection was also performed by Stein and Leventhal for treatment of this endocrinopathy which resulted in resumption of ovulatory menstrual cycle. PCOS presents with a wide spectrum of manifestation ranging from mild menstrual dysfunction to severe disorder of reproductive and metabolic function. The heterogenous clinical presentation and unknown etiology makes this disease a gynecological curiosity with controversial diagnostic criteria and multiple modalities of management.[3]

SYMPTOMATOLOGY

The common clinical features of women with PCOS are menstrual irregularity, signs of hyperandrogenism, infertility, metabolic and psychosexual disturbances.

1. Ovulatory Dysfunction

Menstrual irregularity is seen in the form of oligomenorrhea which gradually progresses to amenorrhea with severe ovulatory dysfunction. Irregular cycles and ovulatory dysfunction is also commonly seen at pubertal transition and defining abnormality at this stage is challenging. Irregular cycles are defined as:[4]

- Normal in the first year post-menarche as part of pubertal transition
- >1 to <3 years post-menarche: <21 or >45 days
- >3 years post menarche to perimenopause: <21 or >35 days or <8 cycles per year
- >1 year post-menarche >90 days for any one cycle
- Primary amenorrhea by age 15 or > 3 years post-thelarche (breast development)

Adolescents with features of PCOS but who do not meet the diagnostic criteria should be considered at risk and a full reassessment advised 8 years post-menarche.[5] Anovulation and excess of estrogen exposure causes endometrial hyperplasia that can cause abnormal and heavy menstrual bleeding. Adolescent girls often present peripubertally and after periods of weight gain with irregular menstrual cycle. Ovulatory dysfunction can exist even with regular menstrual cycles and if anovulation is suspected, serum progesterone levels can be measured.[5]

2. Hyperandrogenism

One of the key diagnostic feature of PCOS is hyperandrogenism affecting between 60 and 100% of patients with this condition.[5] Clinical signs of hyperandrogenism commonly seen in PCOS are hirsutism, acne and androgenic alopecia. If clinical signs are unclear or absent, biochemical assessment is warranted to establish diagnosis or classify phenotype. Hirsutism is the excess growth of coarse, pigmented terminal hair in male pattern distribution like upper lip, chin, chest, midline abdomen, thighs, upper and lower back and upper arms. The modified Ferriman-Gallway (mFG) score is a visual assessment tool to grade hirsutism in which nine masculine body areas are assessed for terminal hair and scored from zero (no terminal hair) to four (terminal hair as in a fully developed male).[6,7] Recent studies have suggested that mFG score of >3 in White and Black women and >5 in Mongoloid Asian women represent true abnormality and hence the recent European Society of Human Reproduction and Embryology (ESHRE) guideline has recommended cut offs of ≥4–6 on mFG for defining hirsutism.[5,8,9] The vast majority (>70%) of women with hirsutism have elevated androgen levels.[10] The degree and distribution of alopecia can be assessed by the Ludwig visual score but there is no universally accepted assessment method for scoring acne.[10] Clinical hyperandrogenism has considerable impact on quality of life and the treatment burden can be significant for patients. Virilization is rare and signs such as deepening of voice, clitoromegaly, increased muscle mass, decreased breast mass indicate severe androgen excess. This warrants exclusion of other conditions like androgen secreting tumor.

3. Infertility

Women with this syndrome have a higher risk of infertility due to oligo-/anovulatory dysfunction. Other mechanisms for the decline in fertility being defective oocyte competence, obesity and unfavorable endometrial changes.[11]

4. Metabolic Syndrome

PCOS is more commonly seen in women who are overweight or obese and particularly have increased visceral adiposity.[12] Obesity increases the risk of insulin resistance, impaired glucose tolerance, diabetes mellitus and metabolic syndrome.[13] Obesity particularly abdominal adiposity decreases sex hormone binding globulin and increases free androgens causing a relative hyperandrogenemia.[14] It has also been demonstrated in meta-analysis that most women with PCOS have hyperinsulinemia and insulin resistance independent of body mass index.[15] PCOS women have 3-fold higher prevalence of impaired glucose tolerance and 7.5–10-fold higher prevalence of undiagnosed type 2 DM.[16,17] This further increases in presence of family history of diabetes.[18] Cardiovascular risk factors are also increased in women with PCOS putting them at higher risk of hypertension and coronary heart disease.[18] Dyslipidemia in the form of increased triglyceride and low density lipoprotein and reduced high density lipoprotein is also seen in PCOS irrespective of BMI.[19] Therefore, all women with PCOS should have regular monitoring for weight, blood pressure, BMI, waist circumference and overweight or obese women should have a fasting lipid profile at diagnosis.[5] Obstructive sleep apnea is also commonly seen in PCOS women especially obese PCOS and insulin resistance is an important predictor.[21]

5. Psychosexual Dysfunction

The prevalence and severity of depression and anxiety symptoms are higher in PCOS patients and routine screening for these symptoms is recommended.[5] Factors like obesity, hirsutism, infertility and hormonal medications in PCOS may independently exacerbate distress and affect emotional well-being. Sexual dysfunction is commonly seen in women with PCOS and they report lower sexual self-worth and sexual satisfaction.[22]

Health-related quality of life in PCOS patients is affected by a multitude of clinical features like anxiety and depressive symptoms, low self-esteem, negative body image, delayed diagnosis and inadequate education and counselling by health professionals.[23] There are tools like PCOS quality of life tool to evaluate symptoms that cause greatest distress to PCOS patients and response to treatment.[24]

Definition: Changing Concepts

It has long been recognized that the basic defect in women with PCOS is hyperandrogenism and a large proportion of women have underlying insulin resistance. Consensus on the defining criteria of PCOS is yet to be reached despite multiple workshops and meetings by professional organizations.

The National Institute of Health (NIH) in 1990 proposed the following criteria for diagnosing PCOS:[25]

a. Chronic oligo-/anovulation

b. Clinical and/or biochemical signs of hyperandrogenism

c. Exclusion of other causes of hyperandrogenism such as androgen-secreting tumors, congenital adrenal hyperplasia, Cushing's syndrome and hyperprolactinemia

Polycystic ovaries on USG may or may not be present and was not included in the diagnostic criteria. In this definition, it was emphasized that the presence of enlarged polycystic ovaries was neither essential nor mandatory for the diagnosis of PCOS and it was primarily considered an ovarian androgen excess disorder.

Clinical signs of androgen excess are the presence of hirsutism, acne or male pattern balding. Where clinical signs of hyperandrogenism (particularly hirsutism) is unclear or absent, it is useful to assess for biochemical androgen excess.[5] Biochemical hyperandrogenism is influenced by the type of androgens measured, the assay method used and cost issues. Total testosterone will identify only 20–30% of women with PCOS having hyperandrogenism whereas free testosterone will identify 50–60%.[5] Free testosterone, free androgen index (FAI = 100 × Total testosterone SHBG) and calculated bioavailable testosterone should be used to diagnose PCOS.[26] Assessment of androgen status should be done in early follicular phase as testosterone secretion increases during mid-cycle and morning levels are most predictive. There is limited role for measurement of androstenedione and dehydroepiandrosterone sulfate (DHEAS) when testosterone levels are not elevated and for exclusion of other causes of hyperandrogenism. Mild elevation of DHEAS may be seen in PCOS, but if significantly elevated or signs of virilization require exclusion of androgen secreting adrenal tumor. Androstenedione elevation is seen in 21 hydroxylase deficient non classical CAH. Hormonal contraception can alter the levels of androgens hence assessment should be done after withdrawing medication for three or more months.[5]

This definition was further modified in a consensus meeting held at Rotterdam in 2003 in which members from ESHRE and American Society of Reproductive Medicine (ASRM) participated.[27] The revised definition expanded the NIH criteria to incorporate a wider spectrum of PCOS phenotypes. After exclusion of other androgen excess disorder, two out of three criteria are essential for making a diagnosis:

a. Oligo- and/or anovulation

b. Clinical and/or biochemical signs of androgen excess

c. Polycystic ovarian morphology (PCOM) by ultrasonography

Polycystic ovaries in the Rotterdam criteria required the presence of 12 or more follicles measuring 2–9 mm in both ovaries, stromal echogenicity or an ovarian volume ≥ 10 cm^3. Recent evidence suggests that the correlation between PCOM and menstrual dysfunction is poor in adolescence as majority have polycystic ovaries on USG. Hence USG should not be used for diagnosis in adolescents less than 8 years after menarche.[28] The threshold of PCOM has also been recently revised with advancing USG technology. When using endovaginal ultrasound transducers of 8 MHz frequency, the threshold for PCOM is defined as on either ovary, a follicle number per ovary of ≥20 and/or an ovarian volume ≥10 mL, ensuring the absence of dominant follicles, corpora lutea or cysts.[5] If using older technology or transabdominal USG, the threshold for PCOM should be an ovarian volume ≥10 mL on either ovary.[5] Therefore, in patients with irregular menstrual cycle and hyperandrogenism, an ovarian USG is not necessary for making a diagnosis but it will help in identifying the complete phenotype. The Rotterdam criteria increased both the prevalence of PCOS as well as variability of phenotype.

Some authors have raised controversy on the Rotterdam criteria because according to this criteria, there will be a group of patients without hyperandrogenism. The delayed consequences of this syndrome that is the metabolic complications are thought to be due to hyperandrogenism and, therefore, this group of patients should not have these complications. They also suggested that this group of patients require further investigation for inclusion in PCOS. According to them, the current definition needs further clarification and modification.[29,30]

The Androgen Excess and PCOS (AE-PCOS) group in 2006 recommended the presence of all the three features for diagnosing PCOS.[31,32]

- Signs of hyperandrogenism (clinical and/or biochemical)
- Ovulatory dysfunction (oligo-/anovulation and/or polycystic ovarian morphology on USG)
- Exclusion of other causes of hyperandrogenism

The NIH held an evidence-based methodology workshop of PCOS in 2012 wherein they suggested the Rotterdam criteria as acceptable for defining PCOS after evaluating different aspects as it is inclusive of both the NIH and the AE-PCOS criteria.[33] The core diagnostic criteria of PCOS was reinforced to include: (1) clinical/biochemical hyperandrogenism (HA), (2) chronic ovulatory dysfunction (OD), and (3) polycystic ovarian morphology (PCOM). They broadened ovulatory dysfunction to include not only oligo-/anovulation but also polymenorrhea and abnormal uterine bleeding. They also suggested an alternate classification of PCOS which categorises women in four different phenotypes. ESHRE in 2018 has endorsed the NIH recommendation that specific phenotypes should be reported in all clinical classification and epidemiological research.[5,33] The four phenotypes are:

1. Androgen excess + ovulatory dysfunction + polycystic ovarian morphology (phenotype A)
2. Androgen excess + ovulatory dysfunction (phenotype B)
3. Androgen excess + polycystic ovarian morphology (phenotype C)
4. Ovulatory dysfunction + polycystic ovarian morphology (phenotype D)

Lizneva, et al. refined the phenotypic approach and proposed three PCOS phenotypes: 'Classic' PCOS (phenotypes A/B), 'Ovulatory PCOS' (phenotype C), and 'Non-hyperandrogenic PCOS' (phenotype D).[34] More than two-thirds women diagnosed with PCOS belonged to the classic phenotype. The classic PCOS compared to other phenotypes had more severe symptoms and were also at significant risk of long-term complications such as obesity, higher rates of insulin resistance and dyslipidemia. The ovulatory phenotype had intermediate severity of symptoms and long-term complications and the non-hyperandrogenic were the least severe. This classification system more accurately represents the PCOS spectrum and will help in more specific patient counselling regarding severity of long-term health risks.[34]

CONCLUSION

PCOS is a heterogenous condition with a wide spectrum of clinical features and long-term health risks. The etiology is unclear but a combination of genetic, environmental and metabolic factors may play a role. Disordered ovarian androgen production leads to an excess of testosterone over estrogens. Hyperandrogenism is an important characteristics of PCOS and is determinant of long-term metabolic complications. The recent phenotypic classification based on Rotterdam criteria has enabled better grading of severity and uniform classification in epidemiological research. Diagnosis of PCOS in adolescents is challenging because of immaturity of hypothalamo-pituitary-ovarian axis and multifollicular ovaries similar to PCOM normally seen in adolescents.

REFERENCES

1. Consensus on women's health aspects of polycystic ovary syndrome (PCOS). Hum Reprod 2012;27(1):14–24.
2. Stein I, Leventhal M. Amenorrhea associated with bilateral polycystic ovaries. Am J Obstet Gynecol 1935;29:181–89.
3. Homburg R. Polycystic ovary syndrome-from gynaecological curiosity to multisystem endocrinopathy. Hum Reprod Oxf Engl. 1996 Jan; 11(1):29–39.
4. Witchel SF, Oberfield S, Rosenfield RL, Codner E, Bonny A, Ibáñez L, et al. The Diagnosis of Polycystic Ovary Syndrome during Adolescence. Horm Res Paediatr 2015;83:376–389.
5. International evidence-based guideline for the assessment and management of polycystic ovary syndrome (PCOS). ESHRE 2018. https://www.eshre.eu/Guidelines-and- Legal/ Guidelines / Polycystic - Ovary-Syndrome.aspx
6. Ferriman D, JD Gallwey. Clinical assessment of body hair growth in women. J Clin Endocrinol Metab. 1961;21:1440–7.
7. Yildiz BO, Bolour S, Woods K, Moore A, Azziz R. Visually scoring hirsutism. Hum Reprod Update. 2010;16(1):51–64.
8. DeUgarte CM, Woods KS, Bartolucci AA, Azziz R. Degree of facial and body terminal hair growth in unselected black and white women:toward a populational definition of hirsutism. J Clin Endocrinol Metab, 2006;91(4):1345–50.
9. Zhao X1, Ni R, Li L, Mo Y, Huang J, Huang M et al. Defining hirsutism in Chinese women: a cross-sectional study. Fertil Steril 2011;96(3):792–96.
10. Lizneva D1, Gavrilova-Jordan L2, Walker W2, Azziz R, et al. Androgen excess: Investigations and management. Best Pract Res Clin Obstet Gynaecol, 2016;37:98–118.
11. Wood JR, Dumesic DA, Abbott DH, Strauss JF 3rd. Molecular abnormalities in oocytes from women with polycystic ovary syndrome revealed by microarray analysis. J Clin Endocrinol Metab 2007;92(2):705–13.
12. Conway GS, Dewailly D, Diamanti-Kandarakis E, Escobar-Morreale HF, Franks S, Gambineri A, et al. The polycystic ovary syndrome: an endocrinological perspective from the European Society of Endocrinology. Eur J Endocrinol 2014;171(4):489–98.
13. Gambineri A, Pelusi C, Vicennati V, Pagotto U, Pasquali R. Obesity and the polycystic ovary syndrome. Int J Obes Relat Metab Disord. 2002; 26:883–896.
14. Pasquali R. Obesity and androgens: facts and perspectives. Fertil Steril. 2006;85:1319–1340.
15. Cassar S, Misso ML, Hopkins WG, Shaw CS, Teede HJ, Stepto NK. Insulin resistance in polycystic ovary syndrome: a systematic review and meta-analysis of euglycaemic-hyper-insulinaemic clamp studies. Human Reproduction. 2016;31(11):2619–2631.
16. Legro RS, Kunselman AR, Dodson WC, Dunaif A. Prevalence and predictors of risk for type 2 diabetes mellitus and impaired glucose tolerance in polycystic ovary syndrome: a prospective, controlled study in 254 affected women. J Clin Endocrinol Metab 1999;84(1):165–69.
17. Ehrmann DA, Barnes RB, Rosenfield RL, Cavaghan MK, Imperial J. Prevalence of impaired glucose tolerance and diabetes in women with polycystic ovary syndrome. Diabetes Care 1999;22(1):141–6.
18. Ehrmann DA, Kasza K, Azziz R, Legro RS, Ghazzi MN. Effects of race and family history of type 2 diabetes on metabolic status of women with polycystic ovary syndrome. J Clin Endocrinol Metab 2005;90(1):66–71.
19. Wild RA, Carmina E, Diamanti-Kandarakis E, Dokras A, Escobar-Morreale HF, Futterweit W, et al. Assessment of cardiovascular risk and prevention of cardiovascular disease in women with the polycystic ovary syndrome: a consensus statement by the Androgen Excess and Polycystic Ovary Syndrome (AEPCOS) Society. J Clin Endocrinol Metab 2010;95:2038–2049.

20. Talbott E, Guzick D, Clerici A, Berga S, Detre K, Weimer K, et al. Coronary heart disease risk factors in women with polycystic ovary syndrome. Arterioscler Thromb Vasc Biol 1995; 15(7):821–26.

21. Vgontzas AN, Legro RS, Bixler EO, Grayev A, Kales A, Chrousos GP. Polycystic ovary syndrome is associated with obstructive sleep apnea and daytime sleepiness: role of insulin resistance. J Clin Endocrinol Metab 2001;86(2): 517–20.

22. Elsenbruch, S, Hahn S, Kowalsky D, Offner AH, Schedlowski M, Mann K, et al. Quality of life, psychosocial well-being, and sexual satisfaction in women with polycystic ovary syndrome. J Clin Endocrinol Metab 2003;88(12):5801–5807.

23. Deeks, A, M. Gibson-Helm, and H. Teede. Is having polycystic ovary syndrome (PCOS) a predictor of poor psychological function including depression and anxiety. Hum Reprod. 2011 Jun;26(6):1399–1407.

24. Jones, G.L, Benes K, Clark TL, Denham R, Holder MG, Haynes TJ et al. The Polycystic Ovary Syndrome Health-Related Quality of Life Questionnaire (PCOSQ): a validation. Hum Reprod 2004. 19(2):371–77.

25. Zawadski JK, Dunaif A. Diagnostic criteria for polycystic ovary syndrome: towards a rational approach. In: Dunaif A, Givens JR, Haseltine FP, Merriam GR, editors. Polycystic Ovary Syndrome. Boston: Blackwell Scientific Publications; 1992. pp. 377–384.

26. Vermeulen A, L. Verdonck, and J. Kaufman. A critical evaluation of simple methods for the estimation of free testosterone in serum. J Clin Endocrinol Metab 1999;84(10):3666–3672.

27. Rotterdam ESHRE/ASRM-Sponsored PCOS Consensus Workshop Group, authors. Revised 2003 consensus on diagnostic criteria and long-term health risks related to polycystic ovary syndrome. Fertil Steril 2004;81:19–25.

28. Kristensen S, Ramlau-Hansen CH, Ernst E, Olsen SF, Bonde JP, Vested A, et al. A very large proportion of young Danish women have polycystic ovaries: is a revision of the Rotterdam criteria needed? Hum Reprod 2010;25(12): p. 3117–3122.

29. Franks S. Controversy in clinical endocrinology: diagnosis of polycystic ovarian syndrome: in defense of the Rotterdam criteria. J Clin Endocrinol Metab 2006 Mar;91(3):786–9.

30. Azziz R, Woods KS, Reyna R, Key TJ, Knochenhauer ES, Yildiz BO. The prevalence and features of the polycystic ovary syndrome in an unselected population. J Clin Endocrinol Metab 2004 Jun;89(6):2745–9.

31. Azziz R, Carmina E, Dewailly D, Diamanti-Kandarakis E, Escobar-Morreale HF, Futterweit W et al. The Androgen Excess and PCOS Society criteria for the polycystic ovary syndrome: the complete task force report. Fertil Steril 2009; 91(2):456–88.

32. Azziz R, Carmina E, Dewailly D, Diamanti-Kandarakis E, Escobar-Morreale HF, Futterweit W et al. Position statement: Criteria for defining polycystic ovary syndrome as a predominantly hyperandrogenic syndrome: An androgen excess society guideline. J Clin Endocrinol Metab 2006;91; 4237–45.

33. NIH Evidence based workshop panel, NIH Evidence based workshop on Polycystic Ovary Syndrome. http://prevention.nih.gov/workshops/2012/pcos/resources.aspx., 2012.

34. Lizneva D, Suturina L, Walker W, Brakta S, Gavrilova-Jordan L, Azziz R. Criteria, prevalence, and phenotypes of polycystic ovary syndrome. Fertil Steril 2016;106;6–15.

11

Polycystic Ovary Syndrome (PCOS) in Adolescents

Sujata Sharma, Garima Sharma, Amarjeet Kaur

Polycystic ovary syndrome (PCOS) is the most common endocrine disorder in women of reproductive age group.[1] It affects 6–15% of women of reproductive age group and 0.5–3% of adolescents. It accounts for 72–84% of cases of hyperandrogenism in adults.[2–4] It is the cause of significant morbidity that includes impaired reproductive health, metabolic syndrome and increased risk of certain cancers. The salient features of this disorder are menstrual irregularities, elevated androgens and polycystic appearing ovaries.

The cause of PCOS is not known and the pathogenesis is not well understood. It is likely a complex interaction between genetic, epigenetic factors, environmental factors, insulin resistance and alterations in steroid metabolism.[5,6] There are variations in symptoms of PCOS with age, weight, race and various medications. Diagnostic problems arise in the adolescents due to an overlap of clinical features of PCOS and characteristics of normal puberty. The purpose of this chapter is to offer understanding and approach to the diagnosis and treatment of PCOS in adolescents.

PHYSIOLOGY OF NORMAL PUBERTY

Puberty is initiated with the maturation of the hypothalamic-pituitary-ovarian axis and secretion of the gonadotropin-releasing hormone (GnRH), the activity of which is suppressed during childhood. Varying GnRH pulse frequencies trigger the pituitary to release LH and FSH, which stimulate ovarian theca and granulosa cells, respectively. Theca cells produce androstenedione, which gets aromatized into estradiol in the nearby granulosa cells resulting in the physiological changes of puberty, i.e. breast development, bone growth, and fat deposition. The adrenal gland also releases increasing amounts of androgens, such as dehydroepiandrosterone (DHEA) and DHEA sulfate, which are responsible for the development of pubic and axillary hair, as well as acne. The subsequent increase in ovarian androgens also facilitates the development of sexual hair.

PATHOPHYSIOLOGY OF PCOS IN ADOLESCENTS

PCOS is a complex disorder arising from genetic and environmental influences. Various possible etiologies include disordered neuroendocrine gonadotropin secretion, hyperandrogenism, obesity, insulin resistance, and hyperinsulinemia or the combination of these factors.[7] Ovarian hyperandrogenism is proposed to be the primary dysfunction in the pathophysiology of PCOS.

Hyperandrogenemia and PCOS

Increased androgen levels, primarily produced by the ovaries (with a smaller contribution from the adrenals and peripheral adipose tissue), interfere with hypothalamic sensitivity to negative feedback from the ovary, thereby increasing GnRH pulse frequency.[7] This persistently rapid pulse frequency favors increased LH secretion, which in turn stimulates the ovarian theca cells to produce more androgens. The relative decrease in FSH secretion leads to less aromatization of androgens to estradiol which leads to impaired follicular development, hence oligomenorrhea and polycystic ovaries.

Androgens also influence the distribution of fat in the body. There is a more visceral distribution of adipose tissue (AT) and these patients have more upper body fat distribution similar to that of men. This different AT distribution is due to the influence of steroids, their metabolism and the expression of tissue-specific steroid receptors.[8,9] This visceral fat is biologically active which further contributes to the metabolic and endocrine disturbances in PCOS resulting in impaired glucose metabolism and insulin resistance.

Catecholamine-induced lipolysis is higher in visceral fat than subcutaneous fat. This may be due to decreased expression of β2-adrenoceptors and hormone-sensitive lipase in subcutaneous fat leading to low lipolysis in this compartment. There is an accumulation of fat in the visceral compartment in spite of the fact that lipolysis in this compartment is higher than in subcutaneous fat. This is possible when rates of fat deposition are higher than the rates of fat mobilization. Dicker et al. proposed that increased lipolysis is important in the development of insulin resistance (IR) in PCOS.[10] Excess free fatty acids derived from lipolysis of acylglycerol in adipocytes accumulate in the hepatic portal veins which leads to hepatic dysfunction, hence elevated glucose secretion. This further leads to increased insulin secretion from pancreas and glucose uptake in AT, thus contributing to development of insulin resistance.

Adolescent Obesity and PCOS

Excess abdominal fat initiates metabolic and endocrine disturbances contributing to the progression of hyperandrogenism. Abdominal AT leads to impaired insulin action as explained above, resulting in further progression of hyperandrogenism. Excessive androgen levels in PCOS lead to impaired glucose uptake, insulin resistance and increased deposition of visceral fat. The complex metabolic inter-relationship between obesity and PCOS has not fully understood yet, but the co-occurrence of both these conditions in adolescents increases the severity of negative health consequences of these conditions.

Hyperandrogenemia and Insulin Resistance (IR)

It was found in various studies that androgens induce IR through activation of androgen receptors in the subcutaneous adipocytes. The effect of insulin on glucose metabolism was impaired due to defects in phosphorylation of a downstream protein, protein kinase-Cζ, which normally mediates the effect of insulin on glucose transport.[11] As a consequence, insulin-stimulated glucose transport was impeded leading to development of insulin resistance. It was also found that the adipocytes from women with PCOS displayed enhanced glycogen synthase kinase-3β (GSK-3β) action. Overexpression of GSK-3β promoted androgen biosynthesis through direct stimulation of P450c17 enzyme activity. Results from these studies illustrated that continuous exposure to androgens led to impairment of insulin action and development of IR.[11,12]

Hyperinsulinemia (HI) and Hyperandrogenemia (HA)

HI contributes to HA by the direct stimulation of steroidogenesis in ovarian theca and granulosa cells. Excess insulin also stimulates hypothalamic GnRH secretion and, therefore, induces gonadotropin secretion particularly LH from pituitary cells, which in turn stimulates androgen production in the ovaries. Lack of FSH decreases aromatization of androgens to estradiol in granulosa cells, thereby interfering with the development of dominant follicle which then leads to polycystic ovaries. HI also decreases sex hormone binding globulin (SHBG) which further worsens hyperandrogenemia. Insulin resistance also promotes the release of nonesterified fatty acids from the liver and adipose tissue due to decreased activity of lipoprotein lipase contributing to dyslipidemia associated with PCOS.

Role of Immunology in the Pathophysiology of PCOS

Obesity has recently been considered as a state of low grade inflammation due to excessive production of cytokines, adipokines and other reactants.[13–16] These inflammatory markers include TNF-α, IL-1, IL-6, IP-10, RP, and IL-18. These mediators initiate insulin resistance, type 2 diabetes and other metabolic complications in patients of PCOS. In a study, it was found that the levels of leptin in PCOS patients were elevated, whereas adiponectin levels were unchanged or lowered.[17] As leptin stimulates gonadotropin secretion that relates to early puberty seen in PCOS and obese girls. Adiponectin is related to insulin sensitivity and lowered adiponectin concentration in PCOS patients is related to insulin resistance. High molecular weight (HMW) adiponectin has an inverse relation with IR and the inflammatory state from abdominal obesity. HMW adiponectin is lowered in women with PCOS.

Women with PCOS have increased levels of CRP compared to healthy subjects.[18,19] These high levels of C-reactive protein (CRP) are strongly correlated with the increased risk of cardiovascular complications. IL-18 is also associated with metabolic complications and development of insulin resistance.

Inflammation is found in obese as well as non-obese PCOS patients. Women of PCOS with normal weight have a higher fat in the visceral area compared to other parts of the body. This visceral distribution of adipose tissue in non-obese patients is probably a causative factor of low grade inflammation in these patients and corelated to the development of insulin resistance.

During a normal menstrual cycle, estrogen promotes the increased production of IL-6 during the follicular phase, which is later inhibited by progesterone in luteal phase. As the patients with PCOS have low levels of progesterone, leading to increased production of IL-6 and overstimulation of immune system.[20]

Role of Anti-Müllerian Hormone (AMH) and PCOS

There is more number of pre-antral and antral follicles in the polycystic ovary. They produce increased amount of AMH which causes anovulation due to inhibition of FSH by AMH, which normally causes follicular development. Higher the concentration of AMH, more the severity of ovulatory disturbances.[21]

Role of Genetics in PCOS

Genetics also play an important role in the origin of this disease. It has been seen through high familial rates of hyperandrogenism and type 2 diabetes in first-degree relatives of women with PCOS. Zhao et al. found that single-nucleotide polymorphism (SNP) rs13429458 is significantly associated with familial based risk of PCOS. The FTO gene on chromosome 16q12.2 is of particular interest. It is an obesity-related gene and has a strong association with increased BMI, greater weight and T2DM. PCOS women with FTO gene had a greater BMI compared to women without PCOS. Ibanez et al. explained the development of IR regardless of obesity through the 'adipose tissue expandibility' (ATE) hypothesis. According to this hypothesis, fat mass storage capacity is set in early life (age <2 years) and again around puberty (age 10–18 years). This explains why not all obese girls develop androgen excess while others do.[22–24]

Pathophysiology of PCOS

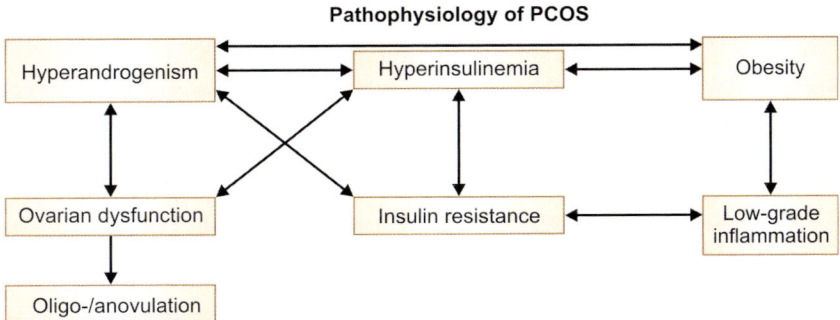

Fig. 11.1: The relationship between various factors involved in the pathophysiology of PCOS

Barker's Hypothesis and PCOS

Although PCOS is familial in majority of cases, various researches led to the 'developmental theory of PCOS' based on Barker's hypothesis. According to this, the offending genes are programmed by excessive *in utero* exposure of androgens. These epigenetic changes in fetal life lead to development of PCOS phenotypes. Various studies implicate that steroidal status of mother permanently alters the physiology of fetus during fetal developmental phase leading to genetic susceptibility to disease after birth. This leads to development of PCOS phenotypes and increased risk of development of metabolic syndrome (type II diabetes and cardiovascular complications). This fetal programming of PCOS traits were experimentally induced in several species by prenatal testosterone exposure.[25]

The summary of the pathophysiology of PCOS is shown in Fig. 11.1.

DIAGNOSIS OF PCOS IN ADOLESCENTS

Since its original description in 1935 by Stein and Leventhal, the definition of PCOS has undergone several changes. Currently, there are three sets of diagnostic criteria for PCOS in adults which are shown in Table 11.1.[26–28]

According to NIH consensus conference held in 1990, PCOS was defined as chronic anovulation with clinical and/or biochemical hyperandrogenism, with the exclusion of other etiologies, such as thyroid disorder or adrenal dysfunction. In 2003, the Rotterdam European Society for Human Reproduction/ American Society of Reproductive Medicine (ESHRE/ASRM) proposed any two out of three criteria consisting of oligo- and/or

TABLE 11.1: Diagnostic criteria of PCOS		
NIH, 1990	*Rotterdam 2003 (ESHRE/ASRM)*	*AE-PCOS Society 2006*
• Ovarian dysfunction[∞] • Clinical and/or biochemical signs of hyperandrogenism (with the exclusion of other etiologies)	• Oligo- and/or anovulation • Clinical and/or biochemical signs of hyperandrogenism • Polycystic ovary morphology[×]	• Clinical and/or biochemical signs of hyperandrogenism • Ovarian dysfunction and/or poly-cystic ovarian morphology
Both criteria are needed for diagnosis	Two of three criteria are needed for diagnosis	Both criteria needed for diagnosis

[∞]Ovulatory dysfunction: Menses are unpredictable and occur at >35 days or occur less than 8 times per year.
[×]Polycystic ovarian morphology (PCOM): >12 antral follicles (2–9 mm in diameter) in either ovary and/or an ovarian volume of >10 mL in one or both the ovaries.

anovulation, clinical and/or biochemical hyperandrogenism, and polycystic ovary morphology (PCOM) on ultrasound; other etiologies must be excluded. The Androgen Excess and PCOS Society (AE-PCOS) 2006 recommends the presence of hyperandrogenism with either menstrual irregularity or PCOM. In December 2012, the NIH's Evidence-based Methodology Workshop on Polycystic Ovary Syndrome supported the broad, inclusionary Rotterdam criteria while specifically identifying the distinct PCOS phenotype shown in Table 11.2.[29]

None of the above groups has proposed different criteria for the diagnosis of PCOS in the adolescent population. There is a debate about the suitability of using these adult criteria in the adolescent population. The use of above adult criteria gives rise to a practical challenge in adolescents because the characteristics of normal puberty often overlap with signs and symptoms of PCOS. In the peri-pubertal period, many adolescents have physiologic menstrual irregularities and signs of hyperandrogenism, e.g. acne. The ovarian morphology also overlaps with that of patients with PCOS in this period. Also, there is no clear description of the normal testosterone levels in this age-group leading to the diagnostic difficulties in adolescents.

Certain metabolic changes that are associated with PCOS are also physiologic during puberty. HI is common in healthy adolescents. Insulin sensitivity decreases by about 50% and there is a compensatory rise in insulin secretion, which later returns to prepubertal levels in adulthood. However, both insulin resistance and HI are more severe in adolescents with PCOS compared with the general adolescent population.

Various adult criteria for PCOS were evaluated in a recent consensus paper of international pediatric and adolescent speciality societies for PCOS diagnosis in adolescents. There was a challenge in differentiating physiological anovulation in adolescents from pathological ovulatory dysfunction. Following criteria were put forth to help in the diagnosis of PCOS in adolescents.[30]

Criteria for Menstrual Disturbances in Adolescent PCOS

This includes any of the following:

- The interval between two consecutive menstrual periods >90 days even in the first year after menarche.
- Majority of adolescents establish a menstrual interval of 21–45 days within the first 2 years after menarche. Menstrual intervals persistently <21 or >45 days 2 or more years after menarche.
- Lack of menses by 15 years or by 2–3 years after thelarche regardless of chronological age.

Criteria of Clinical and Biochemical Hyperandrogenism in Adolescent PCOS

- Persistant increased levels of serum total and/or free testosterone done in reliable reference lab was put forth as best evidence of biochemical hyperandrogenism in adolescent girls with symptoms and signs of PCOS.

TABLE 11.2: Phenotypes in various diagnostic criteria of PCOS

Diagnostic criteria	PCOS phenotypes in various diagnostic criterias
NIH 1990	• AE + OD
Rotterdam 2003/2006	• AE + OD • AE + PCOM • AE + PCOM + OD • PCOM + OD
AE-PCOS society 2006	• AE + OD • AE + PCOM • AE + PCOM + OD
NIH 2012	• AE + OD • AE + PCOM • AE + PCOM + OD • PCOM + OD

All criteria recommend exclusion of other causes of androgen excess. AE, androgen excess; OD, ovulatory dysfunction; PCOM, polycystic ovary morphology; PCOS, polycystic ovary syndrome.

- Hyperandrogenemia is labeled based on the specific testosterone assay used for testing.
- A single androgen level >2 SD above the mean for a specific assay should not be considered to be evidence of hyperandrogenemia in an otherwise asymptomatic patients.
- Moderate to severe hirsutism is considered as clinical evidence of hyperandrogenism whereas isolated mild hirsutism is considered normal in the early post-menarchal years.
- Persistant acne not responsive to topical therapy is considered as clinical evidence of hyperandrogenemia. It should be evaluated for presence of hyperandrogenemia before starting medical therapies.

Criteria for Polycystic Ovary Morphology (PCOM) in Adolescents

- No definite criteria to define PCOM have been established for adolescents. Follicle counts should not be used as a criterion to define PCOM in adolescents.
- Until further studies, an ovarian volume >12 cm^3 can be considered for diagnosis.
- A multifollicular pattern which is defined as the presence of large follicles distributed throughout the ovary should not be considered a pathological finding. It does not have a relationship with hyperandrogenemia and is more common in adolescents.
- In healthy girls with regular menstrual cycles and without hyperandrogenism, PCOM does not indicate a diagnosis of PCOS.
- Abdominal ultrasound in adolescents, particularly in obese girls, may provide inadequate information as TVS is not indicated in adolescents.
- AMH concentrations should not be used to diagnose PCOM.
- It was concluded that ovarian imaging can be delayed during the diagnostic evaluation of PCOS in adolescents until the availability of high-quality data for PCOM.

Other Diagnostic Recommendations

- Other causes of hyperandrogenemia and irregular menstrual periods must be ruled out before the diagnosis is established. Clinicians should remain aware of other possible pathologies such as thyroid dysfunction, elevated prolactin, hypercortisolemia and other causes of virilization which may result in a similar presentation.
- Although obesity, insulin resistance, and hyperinsulinemia are common in adolescents with PCOS, these should not be utilized as diagnostic criteria.
- Insulin resistance and HI can be considered as indications to investigate and treat potential comorbidities.
- A definitive diagnosis of PCOS is not necessary to initiate treatment. Treatment should be initiated even in the absence of a definitive diagnosis as it decreases the risk of future comorbidities.
- Treatment options that both attenuate the current symptoms and decrease the risk for subsequently associated comorbidities are recommended even in the absence of the definitive diagnosis.

EVALUATION OF ADOLESCENTS FOR PCOS

Clinical evaluation includes through history and examination of the patient. The work-up includes both laboratory and ultrasound testing. The lab testing includes S. TSH, S. prolactin, total and free testosterone, DHEAS, 17-OH progesterone; FSH, LH, estradiol in amenorrheic adolescents; and ultrasound of the ovaries. Pregnancy should be ruled out in all cases. Once the diagnosis of PCOS has been established in an adolescent, screening for metabolic abnormalities should be done that includes fasting and 2-hour GTT, lipid profile and fasting insulin.[31, 32]

Measurement of total and/or free testosterone has been the most recommended investigation to document hyperandrogenemia. DHEAS levels are useful for screening primary adrenal source of hyperandrogenemia. ACTH stimulation test should ideally be performed to screen non-classic congenital adrenal hyperplasia (NC-CAH) but this is not practically possible. Instead a morning 17-OHP level of >200 mg/dL should be used as a screening tool for NC-CAH.[33, 34] These hormone levels should preferably be done in the morning. A normal androgen level done during other parts of the day does not exclude hyperandrogenemia. In such cases, repeat morning hormone levels should be drawn, if the patient fulfills the clinical criteria for PCOS.

Generally, pelvic ultrasonography is not recommended for a diagnosis of PCOS in adolescents. However, it should be performed to rule out other pathologies and to exclude androgen producing tumors in all adolescent girls presenting with features of hyperandrogenemia and menstrual irregularities.

METABOLIC RISK IN ADOLESCENT PCOS

Once the diagnosis of PCOS has been established in an adolescent girl, she should be screened for metabolic abnormalities. Metabolic dysfunction is an important risk associated with PCOS and it can manifest at an early age. About one-third of the adolescents with PCOS meet criteria for metabolic syndrome that include obesity, hypertension, dyslipidemia and glucose intolerance compared with approximately 5% of adolescents

from the general population. The increased prevalence of metabolic syndrome at a young age signifies the importance of regular screening of this population to decrease the future risk of diabetes and coronary heart disease.[35, 36]

The 2-hour plasma glucose level after an oral glucose challenge appears is the most reliable screening test for glucose intolerance. The AE-PCOS Society currently recommends all women with PCOS including adolescents should be periodically screened for glucose intolerance using the 2-hour oral glucose tolerance test and complete lipid profile for dyslipidemia.

Obesity is the better predictor of metabolic dysfunction than PCOS status but androgen excess may also increase the risk for metabolic syndrome independent of obesity. It was found in a study that hyperandrogenic subgroups of adolescents with PCOS exhibited the highest degree of insulin resistance and inflammation as compared to non-hyperandrogenic group. Triglycerides and low-density lipoprotein were also higher in hyperandrogenic group as compared with other PCOS sub-group.[37] Therefore, in patients with well-defined hyperandrogenemia, a detailed metabolic work-up should be performed. It is also important to find out the family history for both PCOS and metabolic syndrome as it is a complex genetic disorder with familial clustering.

TABLE 11.3: Pediatric ATP-III criteria of metabolic syndrome

- Blood glucose >100 mg/dL
- HDL-C <40 mg/dL
- Trigycerides >110 mg/dL
- Blood pressure >90th percentile for age and sex
- Waist circumference >90th percentile for age and sex
    - Three out of 5 criteria should be present for the diagnosis of metabolic syndrome.

ATP III, Adult Treatment Panel III; HDL-C, high-density lipoprotein cholesterol

MANAGEMENT

The goal of treatment is to improve quality of life and to prevent both immediate and long-term clinical consequences that include menstrual abnormalities, infertility, the risk of type 2 diabetes mellitus, cardiovascular disease and the development of endometrial hyperplasia and neoplasia. Management include:

1. Lifestyle Modifications

Lifestyle interventions are the first-line treatment for PCOS in obese adolescents.

Weight reduction leads to improvement in menstrual irregularities, decreased metabolic risks and improved androgen excess. Even a small reduction in weight (2–5%) can result in significant improvement in metabolic and reproductive function. The normal weight PCOS patients also benefit from lifestyle interventions. Depression and anxiety are common in PCOS patients. It is important to address these issues and these should be discussed with the patient and their parents. The major challenge in relation to lifestyle treatment is to maintain children/adolescents at a lower or normal weight.[38] Incorporation of moderate exercise into daily activity is essential for maintaining weight loss over longer time.

2. Pharmacological Treatment

Pharmacological treatment may be added to further improve PCOS symptoms like metabolic disturbances, cosmetic issues, and menstrual irregularities to restore fertility. Oral contraceptives and insulin sensitizers (metformin) are currently most commonly used in adolescents with PCOS either in combination with lifestyle interventions or when intervention fails.[39]

Role of Combined Oral Contraceptives (COCs)

COCs are the first choice in the patients with PCOS. The estrogen-progesterone combination suppresses the endogenous HPO axis and thereby interrupts the pathophysiologic mechanism of PCOS resulting in reduced ovarian androgen production. COCs also increase sex hormone binding globulin thereby further decreasing the androgen excess. It is recommended that a progestogen with low androgenic activity should be used in the OCPs. Three commonly used progestogens are cyproterone acetate, drospiernone, and desogestral.

COCs are the first choice for the menstrual irregularities in PCOS. Duration of treatment with COC is not well defined yet, but the improvement is generally noted in the menstrual pattern within 2 to 3 months. As the OCPs have metabolic side effects, this should be kept in mind while treating adolescents who are already at risk of metabolic syndrome.

COCs are also the drug of choice for acne and hirsutism seen in PCOS patients.

Role of Metformin

It has been used in the treatment of metabolic derangements in PCOS, i.e. in patients with glucose intolerance and type 2 diabetes which does not improve with lifestyle changes. It has been shown to regulate HI, reduce the level of androgens, and control the menstrual cycle of women with PCOS. Recently, it has been shown not only to improve metabolic symptoms but also cause a decline in the frequency of certain cancers like breast and endometrial cancers.

It was found in a recent meta-analysis of randomized controlled trials that metformin was as effective as COCs for treating hirsutism. Metformin was found to be superior to COCs for weight reduction and improving glucose intolerance, but COCs were preferred for menstrual regulation.[40]

Role of Other Treatment Modalities

Additional treatment is needed for further improvement of cutaneous symptoms adjunct to COC or metformin. Spironolactone is a potent anti-androgen used in conjunction with COC or metformin. It improves menstrual irregularities and cutaneous manifestations of hyperandrogenism. It does not improve metabolic symptoms. It should be used in combination with effective contraception in sexually active adolescents as it is a potential teratogen. Intermittent low dose finesteride is also effective for the treatment of hirsutism in adolescents with PCOS or idiopathic hirsutism.

Other treatment modalities include cosmetic hair removal, e.g. electrolysis and laser hair removal.

FUTURE PERSPECTIVES IN PCOS

It has been recently postulated that over-exposure to anti-Mullerian hormone while in the womb can be a potential cause of this condition. This was also noticed in a study that the brains of the mouse treated with AMH produce another hormone GnRH in excess. They were treated with a drug that blocks the body from responding to the higher levels of GnRH which led to normalization of symptoms of PCOS in treated mice. This leads to a new way of thinking and open up opportunities for further research.[41]

CONCLUSION

As the more and more numbers of adolescent girls are becoming overweight and obese, they are at potential risk of developing PCOS. The co-occurrence of obesity and PCOS in adolescent girls tends to increase the severity of the negative health consequences of each condition. It is of great importance to detect girls who are obese in adolescence. Counseling and treatment in early stages of the metabolic disturbances may prevent the future adverse effects on their health. One of the most challenging aspects of this syndrome is its ambiguous diagnostic criteria. In the adolescents where the diagnosis is not clear, it is preferable to follow the symptoms and signs and repeat the evaluation in 6 to 12 months. In the future, more research in the genetics and pathophysiology of PCOS is needed to determine preventive risk factors as well as successful treatment modalities for this syndrome.

REFERENCES

1. Fauser BC, Tarlatzis BC, Rebar RW, et al. Consensus on women's health aspects of polycystic ovary syndrome (PCOS): the Amsterdam ESHRE/ASRM-Sponsored 3rd PCOS Consensus Workshop Group. Fertil Steril 2012; 97:28–38. e25. [Pub Med]
2. Nelson VL, Legro RS, Strauss JF, McAllister JM. Augmented androgen production is a stable steroidogenic phenotype of propagated theca cells from polycystic ovaries. Mol Endocrinol 1999;13:946–57.
3. Hashemipour M, Faghihimani S, Zolfaghary B, Hovsepian S, Ahmadi F, Haghighi S. Prevalence of polycystic ovary syndrome in girls aged 14–18 years in Isfahan. Iran Horm Res 2004;62:278–82. [PubMed].
4. Carmina E, Rosato F, Janni A, Rizzo M, Longo RA. Extensive clinical experience: relative prevalence of different androgen excess disorders in 950 women referred because of clinical hyperandrogenism. J Clin Endocrinol Metab 2006;91:2–6.
5. Rosenfield RL. Identifying children at risk of polycystic ovary syndrome. J Clin Endocrinol Metab 2007;92:787–96.
6. Franks S. Polycystic ovary syndrome in adolescents. Int J Obes (Lond) 2008;32:1035–41.
7. Dumesic DA, Oberfield SE, Stener-Victorin E, et al. Scientific Statement on the diagnostic criteria, epidemiology, pathophysiology, and molecular genetics of polycystic ovary syndrome. Endocr Rev 2015;36:487–525. 10.1210/er.2015-1018 [PMC free article] [PubMed] [CrossRef]
8. Blouin K, Veilleux A, Luu-The V, Tchernof A. Androgen metabolism in adipose tissue: recent advances. Mol Cell Endocrinol 2009; 301:97–103.
9. Kuk JL, Lee S, Heymsfield SB, Ross R. Waist circumference and abdominal adipose tissue distribution: influence of age and sex. Am J Clin Nutr 2005;81:1330–34.
10. Dicker A, Rydén M, Näslund E, Muehlen IE, Wirén M, Lafontan M, et al. Effect of testosterone on lipolysis in human pre-adipocytes from different fat depots. Diabetologia 2004; 47: 420–28.
11. Chang W, Goodarzi MO, Williams H, Magoffin DA, Pall M, Azziz R. Adipocytes from women with polycystic ovary syndrome demonstrate altered phosphorylation and activity of glycogen synthase kinase 3. Fertil Steril 2008;90:2291–97.
12. Corbould A. Chronic testosterone treatment induces selective insulin resistance in sub-cutaneous adipocytes of women. J Endocrinol 2007; 192:585–94.
13. Repaci A, Gambineri A, Pasquali R. The role of low-grade inflammation in the polycystic ovary syndrome. Mol Cell Endocrinol 2011;335:30–41. [PubMed]
14. Alexander RW. Inflammation and coronary heart disease. N Engl J Med 1994;331:468–69. [PubMed]

15. Amato G, Conte M, Mazziotti G, Lalli E, Vitolo G, Tucker AT, Bellastella A, Carella C, Izzo A. Serum and follicular fluid cytokines in polycystic ovary syndrome during stimulated cycles. Obstet Gynecol 2003;101:1177–82. [PubMed]

16. Gordon S. Alternative activation of macrophages. Nat Rev Immunol 2003;3:23–35. [PubMed]

17. Lecke SB, Mattei F, Morsch DM, Spritzer PM. Abdominal subcutaneous fat gene expression and circulating levels of leptin and adiponectin in polycystic ovary syndrome. Fertil Steril 2011;95:2044–49.

18. Kelly CC, Lyall H, Petrie JR, JR, Gould GW, Connell JM, Sattar N. Low grade inflammation in women with polycystic ovarian syndrome. J Clin Endocrinol Metab 2001;86:2453–55. [PubMed]

19. Escobar-Morreale HF, Lugue-Ramírez M, González F. Circulating inflammatory markers in polycystic ovary syndrome: a systematic review and metaanalysis. Fertil Steril 2011; 95:1048–58. [PMC free article] [PubMed]

20. Petríková J, Lazúrová I, Yehuda S. Polycystic ovary syndrome and autoimmunity. Eur J Intern Med 2010;21:369–71. [PubMed]

21. Pigny P, Merlen E, Robert Y, Cortet-Rudelli C, Decanter C, Jonar S, Dewailly D. Elevated serum level of anti-Müllerian hormone in patients with polycystic ovary syndrome: relationship to the ovarian follicle excess and to the follicular arrest, J Clin Endocrinol Metab, 2003;88:5957–62.

22. Zhao H, Xu X, Xing X, Wang J, He L, Shi Y, Shi Y, Zhao Y, Chen ZJ. Family-based analysis of susceptibility loci for polycystic ovary syndrome on chromosome 2p16.3, 2p21 and 9q33.3. Hum Reprod 2012;27:294–98. [PubMed]

23. Hannon TS, Janosky J, Arslanian SA. Longitudinal study of physiologic insulin resistance and metabolic changes of puberty. Pediatr Res 2006;60:759–63. [PubMed]

24. Ibáñez L, Lopez-Bermejo A, Díaz M, Suárez L, de Zegher F. Low-birth weight children develop lower sex hormone binding globulin and higher dehydroepiandrosterone sulfate levels and aggravate their visceral adiposity and hypoadiponectinemia between six and eight years of age. J Clin Endocrinol Metab 2009;94:3696–3699.

25. Li Z, Huang H. Epigenetic abnormality: a possible mechanism underlying the fetal origin of polycystic ovary syndrome. Med Hypotheses. 2008;70:638–642. [PubMed]

26. Zawadski JK, Dunaif A. Diagnostic criteria for polycystic ovary syndrome: towards a rational approach. In: Dunaif A, Givens JR, Haseltine FP, Merriam GR, editors. Polycystic Ovary Syndrome. Boston: Blackwell Scientific Publications; 1992. pp. 377–384.

27. Rotterdam ESHRE/ASRM-Sponsored PCOS Consensus Workshop Group, authors. Revised 2003 consensus on diagnostic criteria and long-term health risks related to polycystic ovary syndrome. Fertil Steril. 2004;81:19–25. [PubMed]

28. Azziz R, Carmina E, Dewailly D, et al. Task force on the phenotype of the Polycystic Ovary syndrome of The Androgen Excess and PCOS Society. The Androgen Excess and PCOS Society criteria for the polycystic ovary syndrome: the complete task force report. Fertil Steril. 2009; 91:456–88. [PubMed]

29. National Institutes of Health. Evidence-based Methodology Workshop on Polycystic Ovary Syndrome. 2012. Available online: https://www.nichd.nih.gov/news/resources/spotlight/Pages/112112-pcos.aspx

30. Witchel SF, Oberfield S, Rosenfield RL, et al. The Diagnosis of Polycystic Ovary Syndrome during Adolescence. Horm Res Paediatr 2015. [Epub ahead of print]. 10.1159/000375530 [PubMed] [CrossRef]

31. Escobar-Morreale HF, Carmina E, Dewailly D, et al. Epidemiology, diagnosis and management of hirsutism: a consensus statement by the Androgen Excess and Polycystic Ovary Syndrome Society. Hum Reprod Update 2012;18:146–70. 10.1093/humupd/dmr042 [PubMed] [CrossRef]

32. Rosenfield RL, Helke JC. Small diurnal and episodic fluctuations of the plasma free testosterone level in normal women. Am J Obstet Gynecol 1974;120:461-5. 10.1016/0002-9378(74)90621-8 [PubMed] [CrossRef]

33. Speiser PW, Azziz R, Baskin LS, et al. Congenital adrenal hyperplasia due to steroid 21-hydroxylase deficiency: an Endocrine Society clinical practice guideline. J Clin Endocrinol Metab 2010;95:4133-60. 10.1210/jc.2009-2631 [PMC free article] [PubMed] [CrossRef]

34. Buggs C, Rosenfield RL. Polycystic ovary syndrome in adolescence. Endocrinol Metab Clin North Am 2005;34:677-705, x. 10.1016/j.ecl.2005.04.005 [PMC free article] [PubMed] [CrossRef]

35. Coviello AD, Legro RS, Dunaif A. Adolescent girls with polycystic ovary syndrome have an increased risk of the metabolic syndrome associated with increasing androgen levels independent of obesity and insulin resistance. J Clin Endocrinol Metab. 2006;91:492–497. [PubMed]

36. Alemzadeh R, Kichler J, Calhoun M. Spectrum of metabolic dysfunction in relationship with hyperandrogenemia in obese adolescent girls with polycystic ovary syndrome. Eur J Endocrinol. 2010;162:1093–1099. [PubMed]

37. Fruzzetti F, Perini D, Lazzarini V, et al. Adolescent girls with polycystic ovary syndrome showing different phenotypes have a different metabolic profile associated with increasing androgen levels. Fertil Steril. 2009;92:626–634. [PubMed]

38. Revised 2003 consensus on diagnostic criteria and long-term health risks related to polycystic ovary syndrome. Fertil Steril 2004;81:19–25.

39. Bremer AA: Polycystic ovary syndrome in the pediatric population. Metab Syndr Relat Disord 2010;8:375–394.

40. Al Khalifah RA, Florez ID, Dennis B, et al. Metformin or Oral Contraceptives for Adolescents With Polycystic Ovarian Syndrome: A Meta-analysis. Pediatrics 2016;137. [PubMed]

41. Pigny P, Jonard S, Robert Y, Dewailly D. Serum anti-Mullerian hormone as a surrogate marker for antral follicle count for definition of the polycystic ovarian syndrome, J Clin Endocrinol Metab, 2006, vol. 91(pg. 941–945)

Insulin Sensitizing Drugs in PCOS

Unmesh S Santpur, Priyanka Dahiya

INTRODUCTION

Polycystic ovarian syndrome (PCOS) is the frequently encountered endocrine disorder in reproductive age group of women. The incidence of PCOS is approximately 7%.[1–3] The characteristic feature of this disorder is enlarged and sclerocystic ovary. The patient presents with menstrual disturbances, obesity, infertility and hirsutism.[4,5]

This metabolic disorder may be typically associated with type 2 diabetes mellitus and the metabolic syndrome.[6,7] There is yet another common association of cardiovascular risk factors with insulin resistance (IR),[8] gestational diabetes mellitus (GDM) and pre-eclampsia in affected women.[9–11]

PCOS is one of the leading causes of infertility with anovulatory cycles.

The other metabolic dysfunctions observed with PCOS are:

- Endothelial dysfunction
- Obstructive sleep apnea
- An atherogenic tendency
- Increased occurrence of coronary artery calcification
- Non-obstructive sleep apnea
- Alcoholic fatty liver disease and steato-hepatitis.

Insulin resistance plays a pivotal role in the pathogenesis of PCOS, with compensatory hyperinsulinemia.

Insulin Resistance

It is defined as a reduced glucose response to a given amount of insulin and usually results from defect within the insulin receptor and post-receptor signaling. The IR results in hyperinsulinism as a compensatory mechanism and is thereby implicated in the pathogenesis of hyperandrogenism. The increased levels of circulating insulin has two effects, one being production of increased ovarian androgen and other being decreased hepatic sex hormone-binding globulin synthesis. Thus, bio-availability of the free androgen is enhanced. Consequently, there is premature follicular atresia and anovulation.

When to treat PCOS?

Therapy for PCOS is directed to:

- Treat obesity and associated metabolic complications
- Infertility by ovulation induction
- For cosmetic purpose (i.e. reduction of hirsutism and acne).

Management options in PCOS include:

- Lifestyle modification and weight reduction
- Oral contraceptive pills
- Androgen receptor antagonists
- Insulin-sensitizing drugs (ISD)

Insulin Sensitizers in PCOS

ISD have emerged in a big way as a treatment modality to counteract the IR. Insulin-sensitizing drugs (ISD) are known to attenuate androgenic symptoms in PCOS. Also, they restore ovulation and regularize menstrual cycle and hence reduce reproductive abnormalities.

Classification of Insulin Sensitizers

1. Biguanides—metformin
2. Thiozolidinediones—pioglitazone, rosiglitazone
3. Inositols—myoinositol, D-chiroinositol
4. N-acetylcystiene

1. Metformin

Metformin is a synthetically derived biguanide and is one of the popular oral hypoglycemic, commonly used in diabetes mellitus. The various actions of metformin are reduction in synthesis of glucose in liver, decrease in lipid synthesis, increase in fatty acid oxidation and inhibits gluconeogenesis by reducing gluconeogenic enzyme activities (PEPCK, FBPase, glucose-6-phosphatase). It inhibits hepatic uptake of lactate and alanine also. This results in reduced levels of circulating insulin levels. This is the most desirable effect in PCOS as hyperinsulinism is detrimental to the patient. It does not induce hyperinsulinemia and therefore does not cause hypoglycemia (i.e. has no action on the pancreatic β-cells).

Mechanism of action

The mechanism of action is not exactly clear. It is proposed that it exerts its action on post-insulin receptor, leading to increased glucose uptake by insulin sensitive cells.

Metformin actions

- Decreases gluconeogenesis in liver
- Reduces intestinal absorption of glucose
- Increases insulin sensitivity—enhances peripheral uptake of glucose by the muscles and liver
- Increases uterine vascularization and blood perfusion
- Reduces androgen and LH levels
- Weightloss

Role of metformin in PCOS

- Increases ovulation and pregnancy rates.
- Reduces fasting insulin levels and serum testosterone concentration.
- It has no effect on live birth rates or miscarriage rate.
- Serum lipid profiles are not affected.
- Incidence of twin pregnancy remains unchanged.

Review of literature suggests that the efficacy of metformin in improving the androgenic and metabolic profile in patients with PCOS may be related to:

i. Dosage employed, when metformin is used as the only agent, mandating higher doses.[12–15]

ii. Combination of metformin with other agents viz., estrogen-progestin combination pills or anti-androgenic agents such as flutamide, spironolactone, and cyproterone acetate.[16]

iii. The profile of the PCOS patient, obese or lean and the levels of insulin.[12,14,15]

In the latest Cochrane Review[17] which included 40 studies, with a total of 3,848 women, the average daily dose of metformin was 1500 mg and the study duration ranged from 4 weeks to 60 weeks. No consensus on the dose and duration of metformin therapy was reached.

Women with PCOS who have not responded to clomiphene citrate as first line of treatment, may be offered one of following second-line treatments:

- Laparoscopic ovarian drilling
- Combined treatment with clomiphene citrate and metformin, or
- Gonadotropins

Side effects

- Gastrointestinal
- Lactic acidosis (rare, but serious side effect)
- It is important to screen for chronic renal and liver diseases before starting metformin.

Dose of metformin
- 500–3000 mg/day.

  (Common regimen is 500 mg 3 times a day or 850 mg twice a day).

  Metformin appears to have a limited role in improving reproductive outcomes in women with PCOS, although there may be a benefit to using metformin in specific patient groups, like:
- In obese women
- When combined with clomiphene citrate
- Those with clomiphene citrate resistance
- Those who have been found to have either impaired glucose tolerance or type 2 diabetes mellitus.

2. Thiozolidinediones

Thiozolidinediones (rosiglitazone and pioglitazone) are newer anti-diabetic agents. Thiozolidinediones are selective ligands of the nuclear transcription factor peroxisome proliferator-activated receptor γ (PPAR-γ), which is expressed most abundantly in adipose tissue, but is also found in pancreatic beta cells, vascular endothelium and macrophages.

Mechanism of action
1. Direct action: 'Fatty acid steal' hypothesis, enhances uptake of fatty acid and storage in adipose tissue, resulting in increase in adipose-tissue mass, this spares other insulin sensitive tissues and pancreatic beta cells (from the deleterious metabolic effects of high concentrations of free fatty acids).
2. Indirect action: There is increase in the expression of adiponectin (an adipocytokine with an insulin sensitivity effect) possibly, by reducing the action of enzymes involved in androgen synthesis. It increases insulin action in the skeletal muscle, liver and adipose tissue leading to decreased peripheral insulin resistance.

Thiazolidinediones exert additional benefit in respect to hyperandrogenism, IR, anovulation, and inflammatory mediator levels, in both lean and obese women with PCOS. These advantages are noted, although there is increase in weight, BMI, and waist-to-hip ratio.

Troglitazone was withdrawn worldwide from market 7 years back due to an increased incidence of drug-induced hepatitis.

Rosiglitazone[16, 17]
- Improves insulin sensitivity
- Improves the ovulation rate
- Decreases androgen levels
- Improves menstrual pattern
- Increases BMI

Pioglitazone[18]
- Improves the menstrual pattern
- It has got no effects on
  a. Anthropometric outcomes
  b. Endocrine outcomes
  c. SHBG or metabolic outcomes (fasting insulin)

  There is limited data on the effects of pioglitazone and rosiglitazone in inducing ovulation. These agents are also associated with embryotoxicity in animal studies.

Role in PCOS
- Improves androgen levels
- Improves ovulation rate
- Enhances insulin sensitivity
- No weight reduction

Thiazolidinediones may provide reproductive, metabolic and cardiovascular function benefits to adult women with PCOS in whom previous metformin therapy has failed. Thiazolidinediones remain off-label in adolescents, due to lack of evidence on efficacy and safety.

3. Myoinositol

It is widely distributed in nature; the main source of it is beans, whole grains, nuts and fruits. Myoinositol is absorbed through gastro intestinal tract to an extent of 99.8% and the half life is 22 min. The enzyme, epimerases converts myoinositol to either L or D-chiroinositol. Myoinositol has emerged in the pathogenesis of PCOS and more distinctly in insulin resistance. Inositol belongs to vitamin B complex and is a compound with a formula $C_6 H_{12} O_6$, a sixfold alcohol of cyclohexane. Human adult consumes approximately 1 g of inositol/day in different forms. It is present in the cell membrane. D-chiroinositol (DCI) is inositol compound produced after extensive inositol metabolism.[18]

Myoinositol is a novel method for induction of ovulation in PCOS patients. There are nine possible stereoisomers, of which myoinositol and D-chiroinositol are used as insulin sensitizing drugs in the treatment of PCOS. Myoinositol has a role in the pathogenesis of insulin resistance.

Mechanism of action

- It restores spontaneous ovarian activity and thus fertility.[19]
- It reduces insulin resistance and enhances the ovarian function.

Myoinositol is an important constituent of follicular microenvironment. It plays a significant role in both nuclear and cytoplasmic oocyte development. Inositol 1, 4, 5-triphosphate modulates intracellular Ca^{2+} release. Elevated concentration of myoinositol in human follicular fluid appears to play a role in follicular maturity and provides a marker of good quality oocytes.

Myoinositol therapy acts at different levels. It reduces the amount of FSH required for ovulation. The quality of oocyte is improved by reducing the total amount of germinal vesicles and degenerate oocyte. It also increases the number of oocytes collected after ovarian stimulation in patients undergoing IVF or ICSI.[20]

Myoinositol has a positive influence on insulin plasma levels and it also affects insulin response to oral glucose load. Myoinositol also corrects the hormonal imbalance as it reduces hyperandrogenism as assessed by clinical and biochemical means, by virtue of reduction of plasma insulin levels. It controls lipid and sugar metabolism, stimulates endogenous production of lecithin, and cellular function of nervous system.[20]

Dosage

Two grams twice daily (4 g/day). Treatment regimen is useful to treat all the symptoms and spectrum of PCOS cases and it appears more complete and effective.[19]

Adverse reactions

Myoinositol has a few adverse effects, the majority being gastrointestinal symptoms like, nausea, flatus, loose stools, diarrhea at a dose of 12 g or more.

At 4 g/day, it is completely free from side effects.

Contraindications

It is contraindicated in patients having hypersensitivity to myoinositol product.

Precautions

It should be used with caution in patients suffering from bipolar disorder having hypomanic and manic symptoms.[20]

4. N-Acetylcysteine (NAC)

N-acetylcysteine (NAC) is a stable derivative and an antioxidant of the sulfur-containing amino acid cysteine. NAC is essential for the synthesis of glutathione, which is one of the natural antioxidant and detoxifier.

NAC is a mucolytic and is useful in many respiratory disorders to clear off the secretions. It is prescribed in conditions, such as HIV infection, cancer, cardiac events, smoking, heavy-metal poisoning, and prevention of influenza, epilepsy, and acetaminophen poisoning.

Mechanism of action

- Increase insulin function in the peripheral tissues, i.e. corrects circulating insulin levels and insulin sensitivity
- Improves ovulatory function, folliculogenesis and decline in testosterone levels

- NAC may not completely reverse PCOS manifestations, but ameliorates many of the chief complaints from PCOS. The patient is relieved of the hyperandrogenic effect like hirsutism. The menstrual abnormalities, amenorrhea and dysmenorrhea are reduced. Infertility may be treated and there is an increase BMI.
- Clomiphene citrate has side effects of thinning the endometrial lining which is overcome by NAC.
- NAC reduces insulin resistance, low density lipoproteins, and total cholesterol may help to curb the longer term risks such as cardiovascular diseases.

Actions of NAC
- It is a naturally occurring powerful anti-oxidant.
- It acts on insulin secretion in pancreatic cells and on insulin receptors on human erythrocytes.
- It has antiapoptotic effects
- It can maintain vascular integrity and also said to have immunological functions.

Many mechanisms are proposed to explain the unique action of NAC on ovulation. Borgstrom, et al. demonstrated the insulin-sensitizing activity of NAC.[21] Flughesu, et al. found that NAC caused significant reduction in circulating insulin levels, peripheral IR, serum testosterone levels, and free androgen index in PCOS.[22] Other important mechanisms explaining the beneficial effects of NAC rather than its insulin-sensitizing effects were also reported. Odetti, et al. reported that NAC has antiapoptotic effects on the ovary and apoptosis is definitely responsible for the process of follicular atresia.[23]

Dosage
- 1200 mg of NAC per day.

REFERENCES

1. Franks S. Polycystic ovary syndrome. N Engl J Med 1995;333(13):853–61.
2. Knochenhauer ES, Key TJ, Kahsar-Miller M, Waggoner W, Boots LR, Azziz R. Prevalence of the polycystic ovary syndrome in unselected black and white women of the southeastern United States: a prospective study. J Clin Endocrinol Metab 1998;83(9):3078–82.
3. Diamanti-Kandarakis E, Kouli CR, Bergiele AT, Filandra FA, Tsianateli TC, Spina GG, et al. A survey of the polycystic ovary syndrome in the Greek island of Lesbos: hormonal and metabolic profile. J Clin Endocrinol Metab 1999; 84(11): 4006–11.
4. Stein IF, Leventhal ML. Amenorrhea associated with bilateral polycystic ovaries. Am J Obstet Gynecol [Internet] 1935;29(2):181–91. Available from: http://www.sciencedirect.com/science/article/pii/S0002937815306426
5. Goldzieher JW, Green JA. The polycystic ovary. I. Clinical and histologic features. J Clin Endocrinol Metab 1962;22:325–38.
6. Franks S, Stark J, Hardy K. Follicle dynamics and anovulation in polycystic ovary syndrome. Hum Reprod Update 2008;14(4):367–78.
7. Nelson VL, Legro RS, Strauss JF 3rd, McAllister JM. Augmented androgen production is a stable steroidogenic phenotype of propagated theca cells from polycystic ovaries. Mol Endocrinol 1999;13(6):946–57.
8. Huang A, Brennan K, Azziz R. Prevalence of hyperandrogenemia in the polycystic ovary syndrome diagnosed by the National Institutes of Health 1990 criteria. Fertil Steril 2010; 93(6):1938–41.
9. Kiddy DS, Sharp PS, White DM, Scanlon MF, Mason HD, Bray CS, et al. Differences in clinical and endocrine features between obese and non-obese subjects with polycystic ovary syndrome: an analysis of 263 consecutive cases. Clin Endocrinol (Oxf) 1990;32(2):213–20.
10. Ehrmann DA, Liljenquist DR, Kasza K, Azziz R, Legro RS, Ghazzi MN. Prevalence and predictors of the metabolic syndrome in women with polycystic ovary syndrome. J Clin Endocrinol Metab 2006;91(1):48–53.
11. Hashim HA. Management of Women with Clomifene Citrate Resistant Polycystic Ovary Syndrome–An Evidence Based Approach. In: Mukherjee S, editor. Polycystic Ovary Syndrome. Intech; 2012. page 1–20.
12. Bridger T, MacDonald S, Baltzer F, Rodd C. Randomized placebo-controlled trial of metformin for adolescents with polycystic ovary syndrome. Arch Pediatr Adolesc Med 2006;160(3):241–6.

13. Glueck CJ, Wang P, Fontaine R, Tracy T, Sieve-Smith L. Metformin-induced resumption of normal menses in 39 of 43 (91%) previously amenorrheic women with the polycystic ovary syndrome. Metabolism 1999;48(4):511–9.

14. Nestler JE. Metformin and the polycystic ovary syndrome. J. Clin. Endocrinol. Metab. 2001; 86(3):1430.

15. Morin-Papunen L, Vauhkonen I, Koivunen R, Ruokonen A, Martikainen H, Tapanainen JS. Metformin versus ethinyl estradiol-cyproterone acetate in the treatment of nonobese women with polycystic ovary syndrome: a randomized study. J Clin Endocrinol Metab 2003;88(1):148–56.

16. Tang T, Lord JM, Norman RJ, Yasmin E, Balen AH. Insulin-sensitising drugs (metformin, rosiglitazone, pioglitazone, D-chiro-inositol) for women with polycystic ovary syndrome, oligo amenorrhoea and subfertility. Cochrane database Syst Rev 2012; (5):CD003053.

17. Morley LC, Tang T, Yasmin E, Norman RJ, Balen AH. Insulin-sensitising drugs (metformin, rosiglitazone, pioglitazone, D-chiro-inositol) for women with polycystic ovary syndrome, oligo amenorrhoea and subfertility. Cochrane database Syst Rev 2017;11:CD003053.

18. Galletta M, Grasso S, Vaiarelli A, Roseff SJ. Bye-bye chiro-inositol–myo-inositol: true progress in the treatment of polycystic ovary syndrome and ovulation induction. Eur Rev Med Pharmacol Sci 2011;15(10):1212–4.

19. Unfer V, Carlomagno G, Dante G, Facchinetti F. Effects of myo-inositol in women with PCOS: a systematic review of randomized controlled trials. Gynecol Endocrinol 2012;28(7):509–15.

20. Ciotta L, Stracquadanio M, Pagano I, Carbonaro A, Palumbo M, Gulino F. Effects of myo-inositol supplementation on oocyte's quality in PCOS patients: a double blind trial. Eur Rev Med Pharmacol Sci 2011;15(5):509–14.

21. Borgstrom L, Kagedal B, Paulsen O. Pharmacokinetics of N-acetylcysteine in man. Eur J Clin Pharmacol 1986;31(2):217–22.

22. Fulghesu AM, Ciampelli M, Muzj G, Belosi C, Selvaggi L, Ayala GF, et al. N-acetyl-cysteine treatment improves insulin sensitivity in women with polycystic ovary syndrome. Fertil Steril 2002;77(6):1128–35.

23. Odetti P, Pesce C, Traverso N, Menini S, Maineri EP, Cosso L, et al. Comparative trial of N-acetyl-cysteine, taurine, and oxerutin on skin and kidney damage in long-term experimental diabetes. Diabetes 2003;52(2):499–505.

Role of Statins in PCOS

Pankaj Desai, Munjal Pandya

INTRODUCTION

Polycystic ovarian syndrome (PCOS) is a combination of various symptoms due to an imbalance in hormonal homeostasis. Main features seen in a patient with PCOS are the result of high androgen levels, along with disturbances in lipoprotein equilibrium. Previously known as the polycystic ovarian disease (PCOD), has various pathological changes, thus replacing the word 'disease' with 'syndrome'. Also known as "Stein Leventhal syndrome", it has various defining criteria according to various societies. According to the National Institute of Health criteria, hyperandrogenism and oligo-/amenorrhea are required to stamp a case as of PCOS.[1] Rotterdam criteria consists of fulfilling of any two of three criteria (hyperandrogenism, oligo/amenorrhea, polycystic ovaries).[2] Androgen Access Society (2006) recommended the presence of clinical and/or biochemical hyperandrogenism and either oligo/anovulation or polycystic ovarian morphology.[3] Hormonal profile of PCOS patients has derangements like high androgens, relatively increased estrogens, reduced sex hormone-binding globulin (SHBG), and high insulin levels.

Comorbidities of PCOS

High circulating insulin levels make subjects with PCOS more prone to development of gestational as well as type 2 diabetes. Patients with PCOS are more prone to develop an atherosclerotic disease, as compared to the common population. Low-density lipoproteins (LDL), triglycerides, and very low-density lipoproteins (VLDL) are higher while high-density lipoproteins (HDL) levels are lower in patients with PCOS.[4] The risk of myocardial infarction is more in these patients owing to increased size and stiffness of the left ventricle along with increased homocysteine levels, increased androgen levels and increased chances of calcification of coronary arteries.[3,5] These patients are more prone to develop metabolic syndrome, along with obesity and propensity to develop diabetes.[6]

Chronic anovulation in PCOS patients makes them susceptible to endometrial hyperplasia, which may advance to endometrial adenocarcinoma. PCOS patients have hyperplasia of theca-interstitial cells, caused by increased insulin as well as oxidative stress, leading to hyperandrogenism.[7] It is believed that this increased insulin level is responsible for hyperandrogenism, by increased production from theca-interstitial cells, as well as reduced apoptosis of the same.[8,9] Increased insulin levels also inhibit SHBG, thus increasing unbound free androgen levels.[10]

Oxidative stress has been proved to be instrumental in deranging homeostasis in subjects with PCOS, by increased generation of reactive oxygen species (ROS), which leads to more of systemic inflammation, even in lean patients.[11] Insulin and systemic inflammatory cells are proved to increase oxidative damage independently, inducing theca cell proliferation.[12–14] Oxidative stress also causes disturbances in insulin signalling, thus stimulating more insulin secretion, making it a vicious cycle.

Pathophysiology involved in PCOS has been explained as an algorithm in Fig. 13.1.

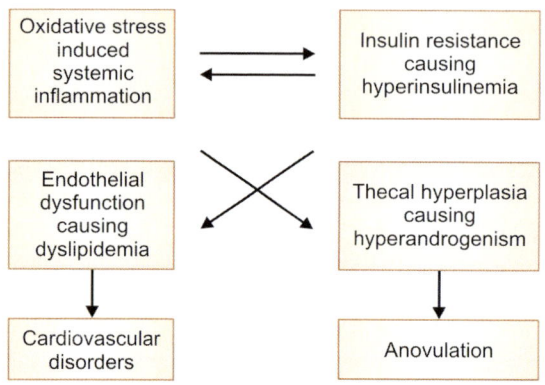

Fig. 13.1: Pathophysiology of PCOS

What are Statins?

Any group of drugs which act to reduce levels of cholesterol in the blood are called statins. They are also known as HMG-CoA reductase inhibitors, are a class of lipid-lowering medications. Also known as hypolipidemic agents, or antihyperlipidemic agents, they are a diverse group of pharmaceuticals that are used in the treatment of high levels of fats (lipids), such as cholesterol, in the blood (hyperlipidemia).

Statins have variety of effects, beneficial for PCOS patients, which include endothelial function improvement, increased nitric oxide, antioxidant effect, reduction in inflammatory markers and immunomodulation. Statins are used for improving lipid profile (reducing LDL), thus will be helpful in PCOS patients. High testosterone levels also decline with their usage, an added advantage offered.[15–18] However; studies have shown little improvement with menstrual irregularity and hirsutism, with statin monotherapy.

Mechanism of Action of Statins

The mevalonate pathway is the all critical pathway in the action of statins. Mevalonate pathway causes the conversion of acetyl-CoA into isopentenyl pyrophosphate, the essential building block of all isoprenoids. It is also known as the isoprenoid pathway or HMG-CoA reductase pathway and is an essential metabolic pathway present in eukaryotes, archaea, and some bacteria. This pathway yields two, five-carbon building blocks called isopentenyl pyrophosphate (IPP) and dimethylallyl pyrophosphate (DMAPP), that are used to synthesize isoprenoids, a diverse class of over 30,000 biomolecules such as cholesterol, heme, vitamin K, coenzyme Q10, and other steroid hormones.

It produces mevalonate from hydroxy-methylglutaryl-CoA (HMG-CoA), the former being an essential product for cholesterol synthesis (Fig. 13.2). The rate-limiting enzyme for this pathway is HMG-CoA reductase, which is reversibly inhibited by statins, thus improving the lipid profile in PCOS patients.[15]

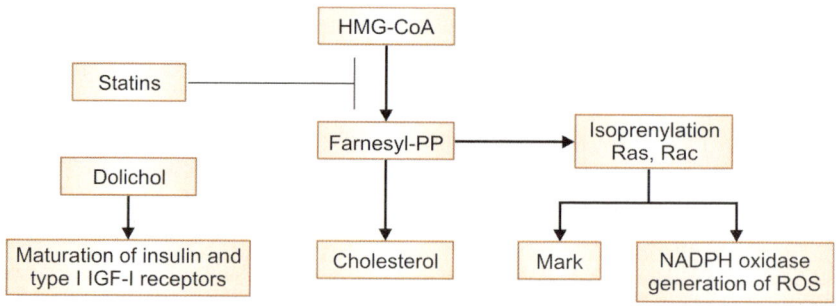

Fig. 13.2: Mechanism of action of statins

Inhibition of this enzyme leads to reduced levels of dolichol, geranyl-geranyl pyrophosphate (GGPP) and farnesyl pyrophosphate (FPP). Dolichol is essential for maturation of insulin and insulin-like growth factor-1 (IGF-1) receptors, so its reduction is helpful for PCOS patients.[19] GGPP and FPP have an important role in post-transitional modification of GTPase proteins, which have an essential role in cellular mechanics.[20] Reduced levels of these proteins, thus, inactivates signal transduction of mitotic activity, decreasing tissue growth, along with a reduction in oxidative stress. The anti-oxidant effect seems to be due to NADPH oxidase activity inhibition as well as inhibition of oxidized LDL production and anti-free radicle action.[21, 22]

Statins are proved to have lowered LDL cholesterol by reducing its synthesis as well as by its clearance, along with improving HDL and triglyceride levels. Inflammatory markers are seen to be reduced as well.[16,17] Statins have been effective in activating AMP-activated protein kinase (AMPK), which is important for cellular metabolic and energy homeostasis.

Hyperandrogenism

Hirsutism is one of the most distressful features, contributing to psychological turmoil of hyperandrogenism. Statins have been promising agents in various studies with a reduction in testosterone level, improvement in LH:FSH ratio, reduction in ovarian size.[23] Cholesterol levels are reduced with statins, which again is a component for androgen production, thus correcting hyperandrogenism.

Polycystic Ovaries

Statins have been effective in reducing the ovarian size, as well as in improving ovarian cycle. Improvement in LH:FSH ratio, along with a reduction in LH level contributes to unifollicular maturation, thus regularizing menstrual cycle. Insulin and IGF-1 actions on the ovary are also limited.

Obesity and Insulin Resistance

PCOS patients usually have impaired insulin sensitivity and statins in a majority of the studies showed a reduction in insulin resistance. Reduced triglyceride leads to more usage of glucose, improving insulin homeostasis. Rosuvastatin showed worsening of insulin sensitivity.[24]

Pre-treatment with atorvastatin, followed by metformin usage, has proved to be of a synergistic effect with improvement in metabolic parameters and inflammatory markers. The study showed that 3 months treatment with atorvastatin followed by 3 months treatment of metformin leads to accumulative 33% reduction in insulin and 35% reduction in HOMA-IR.

Cardiovascular Risk

Improvement in the lipid profile, inflammatory markers with statin usage reduce chances of atherosclerotic risk in PCOS patients.

Clinical Studies

Various studies have been done with statin alone, as well as with oral contraceptive pills (OC pills), with metformin.

Simvastatin

Randomized controlled trials performed with one group on simvastatin with OC pills and the other group on OC pills alone, showed improvement in lipid profile, with reduction in luteinizing hormone (LH) level, testosterone level, inflammatory markers and hirsutism in the former group.[25,26] A trial using metformin, simvastatin, and combination showed the results as reduction in cholesterol was more in patients who received simvastatin (alone and in combination groups), reduction in testosterone was better in simvastatin alone group, improvement in menstrual irregularity was more with simvastatin group.[23] One more study divided patients into two groups, one receiving simvastatin and metformin combination and the other one receiving metformin with placebo. Reduction in testosterone, LDL, total cholesterol, LH, hirsutism was noted in former group.[27]

Atorvastatin

Atorvastatin was found to have reduced inflammatory marker high sensitivity C-reactive protein (hs-CRP), which is a predictor of cardiovascular events.[28] hs-CRP reduction also reduces insulin resistance in pre-diabetics. A trial comparing simvastatin with atorvastatin showed a reduction in testosterone, homocysteine, fasting insulin, LDL and LH levels in both groups. Reduction in homocysteine levels was much greater in atorvastatin group as compared to simvastatin group.[29]

Mevastatin

Mevastatin inhibits theca-interstitial proliferation and androgenesis.[30] Mevastatin has been found to be having an inhibitory effect on mesenchymal cells, including smooth muscle, myocytes, mesangial cells.[31–35] Mevastatin and simvastatin have been found to inhibit NADPH oxidase subunits effectively, thus decreasing steroidogenesis.[36] OC pills have been very promising in improving SHBG when given for at least 3 months, much more effective than statins alone.

Adverse Effects of Statins

Headache, sleep disturbances, drowsiness, nausea, vomiting, abdominal pain, bloating, constipation, skin rash are the known side-effects of statins. Infrequent complications like liver toxicity may occur in patients with acute liver disease. Risk of diabetes may increase and few studies also reported reversible dementia with its usage.[37]

Teratogenesis of statins: Statins have been rated as high-risk category agents, thus making it compulsory for patients to use contraceptive methods along with their use.

Though, statin-induced teratogenicity risk is small.

CONCLUSION

As PCOS is being diagnosed rampantly in today's era, along with lifestyle and dietary modifications. Statins as potentially promising agents need to be given attention for their inclusion in routine usage guidelines, so as to benefit patients with more fruitful outcomes, to their maximum satisfaction.

REFERENCES

1. ACOG Committee on Practice Bulletins-Gynecology. ACOG Committee on Practice Bulletin No. 108: Polycystic ovary syndrome. Obstet Gynecol. 2009;114:936–49.
2. Rotterdam ESHRE/ASRM-Sponsored PCOS Consensus Workshop Group. Revised 2003 consensus on diagnostic criteria and long-term health risks related to polycystic ovary syndrome. Fertil Steril. 2004;81:19–25.
3. Azziz R, Carmina E, Dawailly D, et al. Position statement: Criteria for defining polycystic ovary syndrome as a predominantly hyperandrogenic syndrome: an Androgen Excess Society guideline. J Clin Endocrin Metab. 2006;91(11):4237–45.
4. Rizzo M, Berneis K. Who needs to care about small, dense low-density lipoproteins? Int J Clin Pract. 2007;61:1949–56.
5. Sirmans SM, Weidman-Evans E, Everton V, Thompson D. Polycystic ovary syndrome and chronic inflammation: pharmaco therapeutic implications. Ann Pharmacother. 2012;46:403–18.
6. Apridonidze T, Essah PA, Iuorno MJ, Nestler JE. Prevalence and characteristics of the metabolic syndrome in women with polycystic ovary syndrome. J Clin Endocrinol Metab. 2005;90:1929–35.
7. Nelson VL, Legro RS, Strauss JF, et al. Augmented androgen production is a stable steroidogenic phenotype of propagated theca cells from polycystic ovaries. Molecular Endocrinology. 1999;13(6):946–57.
8. Dunaif A, Green G, Futterweit W, Dobrjansky A. Suppression of hyperandrogenism does not improve peripheral or hepatic insulin resistance in the polycystic ovary syndrome. J Clin Endocrinol Metab. 1990;70:699–704.

9. Nestler JE, Barlascini CO, Matt DW, et al. Suppression of serum insulin by diazoxide reduces serum testosterone levels in obese women with polycystic ovary syndrome. J Clin Endocrinol Metab. 1989;68:1027–32.

10. Nestler JE, Powers LP, Matt DW, et al. A direct effect of hyperinsulinemia on serum sex hormone-binding globulin levels in obese women with the polycystic ovary syndrome. J Clin Endocrinol Metab. 1991;72:83–9.

11. Yilmaz M, Bukan N, Ayvaz G, et al. The effects of rosiglitazone and metformin on oxidative stress and homocysteine levels in lean patients with polycystic ovary syndrome. Hum Reprod. 2005;20(12):3333–40.

12. Adamson GM, Billings RE. Tumor necrosis factor induced oxidative stress in isolated mouse hepatocytes. Arch Biochem Biophys. 1992; 294:223–9.

13. Krieger-Brauer HI, Kather H. Human fat cells possess a plasma membrane-bound H_2O_2 generating system that is activated by insulin via a mechanism bypassing the receptor kinase. J Clin Invest. 1992;89:1006–13.

14. Rifici VA, Schneider SH, Khachadurian AK. Stimulation of low-density lipoprotein oxidation by insulin and insulin like growth factor I. Atherosclerosis. 1994;107:99–108.

15. Kodaman PH, Duleba AJ. Statins: Do they have potential in the treatment of polycystic ovary syndrome? Semin Reprod Med. 2008 Jan; 26(1): 127–138.

16. Sathyapalan T, Atkin SL. Evidence for statin therapy in polycystic ovary syndrome. Ther Adv Endocrinol Metab. 2010;1:15–22.

17. Ferri N, Corsini A. Clinical evidence of statin therapy in non-dyslipidemic disorders. Pharmacol Res. 2014;88:20–30.

18. Raval AD, Hunter T, Stuckey B, Hart RJ. Statins for women with polycystic ovary syndrome not actively trying to conceive. Cochrane Database Syst Rev. 2011;(10):CD008565.

19. Carlberg M, Dricu A, Blegen H, et al. Mevalonic acid is limiting for N-linked glycosylation and translocation of the insulin-like growth factor-I receptor to the cell surface. Evidence for a new link between 3-hydroxy-3-methylglutaryl coenzyme A reductase and cell growth. J Biol Chem. 1996;271:17453–62.

20. Zhang FL, Casey PJ. Protein prenylation: molecular mechanism and functional conse-quences. Ann Rev Biochem. 1996;65:241–69.

21. Wassmann S, Laufs U, Muller K, et al. Cellular antioxidant effects of atorvastatin in vitro and in vivo. Arterioscler Thromb Vasc Biol. 2002;22:300–5.

22. Franzoni F, Quinones-Galvan A, Regoli F, Ferrannini E, Galetta F. A comparative study of the in vitro antioxidant activity of statins. Int J Cardiol. 2003;90:317–21.

23. Banaszewska B, Pawelczyk L, Spaczynski RZ, Duleba AJ. Comparison of simvastatin and metformin in treatment of polycystic ovary syndrome: prospective randomized trial. J Clin Endocrinol Metab. 2009;94:4938–45.

24. Ghazeeri G, Abbas HA, Skaff B, Harajly S, Awwad J. Inadequacy of initiating rosuvastatin then metformin on biochemical profile of polycystic ovarian syndrome patients. J Endocrinol Invest. 2015;38:643–51.

25. Duleba AJ, Banaszewska B, Spaczynski RZ, Pawelczyk L. Simvastatin improves biochemical parameters in women with polycystic ovary syndrome: results of a prospective, randomized trial. Fertil Steril. 2006;85:996–1001.

26. Banaszewska B, Pawelczyk L, Spaczynski RZ, Dziura J, Duleba AJ. Effects of simvastatin and oral contraceptive agent on polycystic ovary syndrome: prospective randomized cross-over trial. J Clin Endocrinol Metab. 2007;92:456–61.

27. Kazerooni T, Shojaei-Baghini A, Dehbashi S, Asadi N, Ghaffarpasand F, Kazerooni Y. Effects of metformin plus simvastatin on polycystic ovary syndrome: a prospective, randomized, double-blind, placebo-controlled study. Fertil Steril. 2010;94:2208–13.

28. Raja-Khan N, Kunselman AR, Hogeman CS, Stetter CM, Demers LM, Legro RS. Effects of atorvastatin on vascular function, inflammation, and androgens in women with polycystic ovary syndrome: a double-blind, randomized, placebo-controlled trial. Fertil Steril. 2011;95:1849–52.

29. Kaya C, Cengiz SD, Berker B, Demirtas S, Cesur M, Erdogan G. Comparative effects of atorvas-tatin and simvastatin on the plasma total homocysteine levels in women with polycystic ovary syndrome: a prospective randomized study. Fertil Steril. 2009;92:635–42.

30. Izquierdo D, Foyouzi N, Kwintkiewicz J, Duleba AJ. Mevastatin inhibits ovarian theca-interstitial cell proliferation and steroidogenesis. Fertil Steril. 2004;82:1193–7.

31. O'Driscoll G, Green D, Taylor RR. Simvastatin, an HMG coenzyme A reductase inhibitor, improves endothelial function within 1 month. Circulation. 1997;95:1126–31.

32. Axel DI, Riessen R, Runge H, Viebahn R, Karsch KR. Effects of cerivastatin on human arterial smooth muscle cell proliferation and migration in transfilter cocultures. J Cardiovasc Pharmacol. 2000;35:619–29.

33. Buemi M, Allegra A, Senatore M, et al. Pro-apoptotic effect of fluvastatin on human smooth muscle cells. Eur J Pharmacol. 1999;370:201–3.

34. El-Ani D, Zimlichman R. Simvastatin induces apoptosis of cultured rat cardiomyocytes. J Basic Clinical Physiol Pharmacol. 2001;12(4):325–38.

35. Danesh FR, Sadeghi MM, Amro N, et al. 3-Hydroxy-3-methylglutaryl CoA reductase inhibitors prevent high glucose-induced proliferation of mesangial cells via modulation of Rho GTPase/p21 signaling pathway: implications for diabetic nephropathy. Proc Natl Acad Sci USA. 2002;99:8301–5.

36. Piotrowski P, Kwintkiewicz J, Rzepczynska I, Duleba AJ. Simvastatin and mevastatin inhibit expression of NADPH oxidase subunits: p22phox and p47phox in rat theca-interstitial cells; 52nd Annual Meeting of the Society for Gynecologic Investigation; Los Angeles, CA. 2005.Mar 23–6.

37. Thompson PD, Panza G, Zaleski A, Taylor B. Statin-associated side effects. J Am Coll Cardiol. 2016;67:2395–410.

Adjuvant Therapy in Polycystic Ovary Syndrome

Ratnakant Talukdar, Madhukar Shinde

Polycystic ovary syndrome (PCOS) is the most common endocrinological disorder affecting young women in the adolescent and reproductive age group. Its incidence has been variously described from affecting 4–12% of women. In India, several studies have shown that the incidence in urban areas may be even more. As development has taken place, the lifestyle diseases are taking upper hand in India surpassing the communicable diseases. PCOS has also been the most controversial medical condition and every aspect has received a lot of attention from the nomenclature, diagnosis and to the management. PCOS is called polycystic 'ovarian' syndrome implying that the primary pathology lies in or triggered by the ovary. It was also called polycystic ovarian disease (PCOD), which is the least used term. Now it has been established that it is actually a part of metabolic syndrome and ovarian pathology is just a reflection of it.

Currently, PCOS refers to being a disorder with a combination of reproductive and metabolic characteristics. This has evolved over time with controversy over the definition culminating in the latest consensus.[1] In the European Society of Human Reproduction and Embryology/American Society of Reproductive Medicine (ESHRE/ASRM) consensus, at least two of the following features are a must to reach the diagnosis;

1. Oligo-/anovulation

2. Hyperandrogenism

3. Polycystic features on ultrasound scan.

The Androgen Excess Society, however, recommended that androgen excess should remain a constant feature of PCOS irrespective of the ovulatory status and morphological features of the ovaries.[2] For almost three decades, PCOS has been regarded as a lifestyle disease which has a long-term impact on the risk of type 2 diabetes mellitus (T2DM) as well as any concomitant cardiovascular disease (CVD) risks besides its reproductive problems.[3]

The problems faced by all gynecologists for PCOS are basically threefold. Young unmarried girls with menstrual problems need a different type of management compared to the married with anovulatory infertility. The older women with metabolic syndrome again are at different risks and consequently require different management.

Although adolescent and young women with PCOS present with obesity, anovulation and insulin resistance, all these may be considered as minor compared to the management of anovulation in the married infertile population. Although various ovulation inducing agents and protocols are available, because of the peculiar nature of metabolic disease these women suffer from, these agents and protocols are less effective than normal women without PCOS. A whole range of additives or adjuvant have been tried with times to make this ovulation induction more effective. These are:

• Lifestyle modification

• Metformin

- Myoinositol
- N-acetylcysteine
- Chromium picolinate
- Vitamin D
- Melatonin
- Glucocorticoids
- Herbal and acupuncture, etc.

LIFESTYLE MODIFICATION

Lifestyle modification has been shown to be the single most effective therapy to control PCOS and improve ovulation and pregnancy rates. Obese women are three times more likely to suffer from infertility as compared to normal weight women. It may be said that 80% of anovulatory infertile women have PCOS. For each unit increase in BMI above normal, there is fourfold increase in the rate of infertility. In case of central obesity, the chance of pregnancy goes down by 30% per cycle for every increase by 0.1 in the waist to hip ratio above normal.[4]

It is interesting to observe that follicular fluid insulin and androgen levels correlate with BMI in obese infertile woman even in absence of PCOS. Higher the BMI, there is that much more circulating androgen which in turn leads to premature follicular atresia and lower follicular maturation causing anovulation.[5] Insulin resistance is present in 50% of PCOS patients, but 90% of obese women have insulin resistance. Insulin resistance again exaggerates ovulatory dysfunction.[6]

There is evidence to prove that as little as 5% reductions in weight lead to ovulation and better pregnancy outcome. Lifestyle intervention in PCOS women improves body composition, hyperandrogenemia and insulin resistance.[7] Lifestyle modification basically consists of diet and exercise and counseling and dedication are both required for it to be successful.

Diet

Obese PCOS patients are recommended diet low in calories with a reduced carbohydrate intake. A loss of at least 5–10% is necessary to re-establish ovarian function in such patients. Nowadays lots of fad diets are available which are either low carbohydrate, low fat ones or low carb-high protein ones. Exceptional diets like extremely high fatty or keto diets are also becoming popular for crash dieting. Diet should be adjusted to individuals keeping in mind the co-morbidities present. Any diet reducing even 5% weight from baseline will lead to menstrual normalcy.

Exercise

Several studies have attempted to establish the role of exercise in the treatment of obese PCOS patients.[8] No significant differences were observed with different diets in association with or without exercise, although a longer weight loss time is often needed in these patients. Increased physical activity is recommended in these patients, although a knowledge gap exists regarding the optimal type, duration, and frequency of exercise.

Bariatric Surgery

Bariatric surgery has recently been advocated as a strategy for weight loss in the morbidly obese patients. If weight loss cannot be achieved with diet and exercise alone, bariatric surgery can be offered. Two primary approaches, restrictive and combined restrictive, and malabsorptive procedures, adjustable gastric banding, and the Roux-en-Y gastric bypass are commonly performed. On an average, bariatric surgery resulted in a loss of 41 ±9 kg in 12 months and improvements in ovulation, insulin resistance, hyperandrogenism, and hirsutism. In a group of 12 PCOS patients available for follow-up after bariatric surgery for morbid obesity, regular cycles were restored in all.[9] Of note, women who have had bariatric surgery are at increased risk for nutritional deficiencies, including protein, iron, vitamin B_{12}, folate, vitamin D, and calcium; however, no consensus exists regarding optimal nutritional screening and supplementation.

Polycystic Ovary Syndrome and Insulin Resistance

Insulin resistance is regarded as failure of the target cells to respond to normal or ordinary levels of insulin. This definition may not be universally agreeable but it gives a simplified understanding of the condition for the purpose of this chapter. Other definitions have been offered by the World Health Organization (WHO). In presence of IR, there is compensatory increased production of insulin by the pancreatic beta cells to control the hyperglycemia, leading to type II diabetes. In PCOS, hyperinsulinemia has been thought to increase hyperandrogenemia via a central role[10] or by decreasing the circulating levels of sex hormone binding globulin.[11]

IR is not considered a diagnostic criterion in PCOS.[1] However, it is recognized by many as a common feature in PCOS independent of obesity.[12, 13] An estimated prevalence of IR among PCOS patients of 60–70% has been reported.[14] However, being overweight or obese is common among PCOS women, affecting up to 88% of these women,[15] therefore, casting doubt on the role IR in the pathogenesis of PCOS. Further, clinical quantification of IR is not accurate enough to enable a better understanding of the role of IR in PCOS pathogenesis or to incorporate it into the work-up program of PCOS patients.[16] However, it is generally acceptable that IR plays a significant role in PCOS either directly or through obesity and represents a clinical concern to physicians and patients.

METFORMIN

Metformin is the only remaining member of the biguanide family that has been used for the treatment of diabetes for a long time. It is the most commonly used drug in T2DM. Metformin works by improving the sensitivity of peripheral tissues to insulin, which results in a reduction of circulating insulin levels. Metformin inhibits hepatic gluconeogenesis and it also increases the glucose uptake by peripheral tissues and reduces fatty acid oxidation. Metformin has a pragmatic effect on the endothelium and adipose tissue independent of its action on insulin and glucose levels.[17]

The main side effects associated with metformin treatment are the gastrointestinal symptoms of nausea, diarrhea, flatulence, bloating, anorexia, metallic taste and abdominal pain. These symptoms occur with variable degrees in patients and in most cases resolve spontaneously. The severity of side effects can be reduced by gradual administration of metformin and titrating the dose increase guided by the severity of symptoms. A starting dose of 500 mg daily during the main meal of the day for 1–2 weeks can lessen the side effects and allow tolerance to develop. A weekly or biweekly increase by 500 mg a day can then be pursued as required until a maximum dose of 1500–2500 mg/day is reached depending on the clinical benefit and side effects. If the dose increase results in worsening of the side effects, the current dose can be maintained for 2–4 weeks until tolerance is developed.[18] Slow release metformin can be associated with fewer side effects. Metformin can also lead to vitamin B_{12} malabsorption in the distal ileum in approximately 10–30% of patients which is an effect dependent on age, dose and duration of treatment.[19] Rarely, lactic acidosis can occur, mainly in diabetic patients, which is a serious condition that can potentially be fatal. Metformin is contraindicated in renal disease as it increases the risk of lactic acidosis.

Metformin in PCOS

The first insulin sensitizing drug (ISD) used in PCOS to decode the role of insulin resistance in the pathogenesis of the syndrome was metformin. Velazquez and colleagues reported in an observational study a significant improvement in menstrual regularity and reduction in circulating androgen levels as well as a significant reduction in body weight which confounded their findings.[20] A few years later, another ISD (troglitazone, which is no longer available) was used in a similar study and reported improvement in cycle regularity and serum androgen levels despite the lack of change in body weight.[21]

Various studies have reported conflicting evidence regarding metformin's status in PCOS. Several meta-analyses that incorporated all of the accessible evidence have also been published with conflicting results.[22]

In principle, ISD works in PCOS by reducing the circulating insulin levels. There is, however, some conflicting evidence as to whether metformin can directly affect ovarian steroidogenesis.[23] Studies have reported many effects of metformin in PCOS patients as; reducing weight, reducing circulating androgen levels, restoring ovulation, reducing the risk of miscarriage and reducing the risk of gestational diabetes mellitus. In IVF, addition of metformin to the ovarian stimulation regime improves the pregnancy outcome.

Metformin and Ovulation Induction

Several of the early studies on metformin in PCOS were compiled in a meta-analysis by Lord and colleagues.[24] It led to conclusion that metformin was effective in inducing ovulation in PCOS patients. It is justifiable to be used as a first-line treatment in conjunction with a change in lifestyle. They included 7 studies comprising a total of 156 PCOS patients who received metformin of whom 72 (46%) ovulated *versus* 1154 who received either placebo or no treatment of whom 37 (24%) ovulated. It was reported that the combination of metformin and clomiphene citrate (CC) resulted in better ovulation rates than CC alone. However, this was based on relatively smaller number of patients included in two and three studies.

Palomba and colleagues, in a meta-analysis, concluded that the combination of metformin with CC is not superior to CC alone in regard to ovulation, miscarriage, pregnancy, or live birth rates.[25] Metformin in combination with CC was more effective in ovulation and pregnancy rates than metformin alone.

It is important to analyse that duration of treatment also plays a role in the outcome. Metformin takes longer to exert an effect in comparison to CC, therefore, CC should be considered the first line of treatment in ovulation induction among PCOS patients. Lifestyle change leading to significant weight loss is an important adjuvant to medications in such patients.

Metformin and IVF

There is a dearth of studies reporting on the use of metformin in conjunction with gonadotropin for ovarian stimulation for the purpose of IVF treatment. A recent Cochrane review has concluded that adding metformin to the ovarian stimulation protocol in PCOS undergoing IVF treatment had no impact on pregnancy or live birth rates. However, it reduced the risk of ovarian hyperstimulation syndrome (OHSS).[26] In a small study, it was reported that the addition of metformin to an antagonist protocol improved the oocyte quality in PCOS patients undergoing IVF.[27] However, a recent Cochrane review revealed that even though metformin was associated with improved clinical pregnancy and ovulation rate, it did not improve live birth rates when used alone or in combination with clomiphene or when compared with clomiphene.[28] Therefore, there is need for developing therapeutic options for treating the women with PCOS.

Metformin and Steroidogenesis

The effect of metformin on androgen production has been controversial. It may be argued that the metformin effect on circulating androgen is a by product of ovulation resumption. However, *in vitro* experiments demonstrated that metformin significantly inhibited both androstenedione and testosterone production by the theca cells.[29] Further, it has been suggested that metformin reduces hyper-androgenism through its effect on both the ovary and adrenal gland suppressing their androgen production, reducing pituitary luteinizing hormone and increases the production of sex hormone binding globulin by the liver.[30] Harborne and colleagues, on the other hand, reported no significant changes in androgen or sex hormone binding globulin levels in hirsute patients treated with metformin and assigned the improvement in symptoms to the reduction of circulating insulin levels.[31] Others reported that reducing fasting insulin and insulin-stimulated glucose levels leads to a reduction in ovarian cytochrome P450c17α activity in obese and lean PCOS patients.[32] A meta-analysis of three RCTs comparing metformin with combined oral contraceptives (COC) on hirsutism gave a no difference verdict.[33]

MYOINOSITOL

Myoinositol (MI) is one stereoisomer of a C_6 sugar alcohol that belongs to the inositol family. It is the precursor of inositol triphosphate, acting as an intracellular second messenger and regulating a number of hormones such as thyroid-stimulating hormone, follicle-stimulating hormone (FSH) and insulin.

Inositol or its phosphates and associated lipids are found in many foods, in particular fruits, especially cantaloupe and oranges. In plants, the hexaphosphate of inositol, phytic acid or its salts, the phytates, serve as phosphate stores in seed, as in nuts and beans. Cereals with high bran content also contain phytic acid. Phytate is not digestible in humans. Food processing techniques to partly breakdown phytates to change this are also available. However, inositol in the form of glycerophospholipids, as found in certain plant-derived substances such as lecithins is well-absorbed and relatively bioavailable.

Myoinositol (phosphate free) was once considered vitamin B_8 of the vitamin B complex. It is produced by the human body from glucose.

MI and D-chiro-inositol (DCI), another stereoisomeric form of inositol, act in different ways to balance some metabolic deregulations concurring with insulin resistance (IR). MI-derived phosphoinositol-3-phosphate (PIP3) enhances glucose transport inside the cells through the stimulation of GLUT4 translocation to the cell membrane. Its derivative inositol phosphoglycan plays a crucial role in downregulating the release of free fatty acids from adipose tissues, hindering the enzyme adenylate cyclase. Indeed, FFA is known to reduce glucose disposal, causing IR and increased triglyceride synthesis. DCI upregulates pyruvate dehydrogenase, leading to the production of ATP by the Krebs' cycle. MI and DCI promote glycogen synthase, inducing glucose conversion to glycogen-stored inside cells. MI modulates the activation of glucose transporters and glucose utilization, and glycogen synthesis takes place under the control of DCI. This molecule on the ovary regulates the insulin-induced androgen synthesis, whereas MI regulates glucose uptake and FSH signalling.[34]

In view of its recognized insulin-sensitizing activity, MI has been used to prevent and/or treat a number of metabolic disorders related to IR, such as the metabolic syndrome, gestational diabetes mellitus and the polycystic ovary syndrome (PCOS).

Myoinositol (MI) supplementation in women with polycystic ovary syndrome (PCOS) has been evaluated over the last years. Many hormonal and reproductive impairments associated with this disorder seem relieved by the supplement. A meta-analysis was conducted by Vittorio Unfer et al with his colleagues from Italy and USA and published in Endocrine Connections in Nov 2017 to assess the effects of MI alone or combined with D-chiro-inositol (DCI) on the endocrine and metabolic abnormalities of women with PCOS. Literature was retrieved from various databases up to 2016. Only randomized controlled trials investigating the effects of myoinositol alone or in combination with DCI were reviewed.[35] Nine RCTs involving 247 cases and 249 controls were included. Significant decreases in fasting insulin and homeostasis model assessment (HOMA) index were identified after MI supplementation. The trial sequential analysis of insulin meta-analysis illustrated that the cumulative z-curve crossed the monitoring boundary, providing strong proof of the intervention effect. A slight trend toward a reduction of testosterone concentration by MI with respect to controls was found, whereas androstenedione levels remained unaffected. Throughout a subgroup's meta-analysis, a significant increase in serum SHBG was observed only in those studies where MI was administered for at least 24 weeks. These results point towards the beneficial effect of myoinositol in improving the metabolic profile in PCOS, concomitantly reducing their hyperandrogenism.

Using a questionnaire, an observational study was performed under German gynecologists[36] to collect data on ovulation and pregnancy rates in PCOS patients with infertility. In this observational study, 3602 infertile women used myoinositol and folic acid between 2 and 3 months in a dosage of 2 × 2000 mg myoinositol + 2 × 200 µg folic acid per day. In a subgroup of 32 patients, hormonal values for testosterone, free testosterone, and progesterone were analyzed before and after three months of treatment. The mean time of use was 10.2 weeks. During this time period, 70% of these women had a restored ovulation, and a pregnancy rate of 15.1% of all the myoinositol and folic acid users occurred. In 19 cases, a concomitant medication with clomiphene or dexamethasone was used. One twin pregnancy was documented. Testosterone levels changed from 96.6 to 43.3 ng/mL and progesterone from 2.1 to 12.3 ng/mL ($p < 0.05$) after 12 weeks of treatment. No relevant side effects were present among the patients. This study could show that a new treatment option for patients with a PCOS and infertility is available. The achieved pregnancy rates are at least in an equivalent or even superior range than those reported by the use of metformin. The use of 2 × 2000 mg myoinositol + 2 × 200 µg folic acid per day is a safe and promising tool in the effective improvement of symptoms and infertility for patients with a polycystic ovary syndrome (PCOS).

N-ACETYLCYSTEINE

Acetylcysteine, also known as **N-acetylcysteine (NAC)**, is used to treat paracetamol overdose, and as a safe mucolytic drug in individuals with cystic fibrosis or chronic obstructive pulmonary disease.[37] It can be taken intravenously, by mouth, or inhaled as a mist.[37] It is also used as a dietary supplement.

Common side effects include nausea and vomiting when ingested orally. There may be reddness and itching over skin with either form. A non-immune type of anaphylaxis, which is safe during pregnancy may also occur. In cases of paracetamol overdose, it works by increasing the level of glutathione, that neutralizes the toxic breakdown products of paracetamol. When paracetamol is ingested in larger quantities, a minor metabolite called N-acetyl-p-benzoquinone imine (NAPQI) accumulates within the body. It is normally conjugated by glutathione, but when taken in excess, the body's glutathione reserves are not sufficient to inactivate the toxic NAPQI. This metabolite is then free to react with key hepatic enzymes, thereby damaging liver cells. This may lead to severe liver damage and even death by acute liver failure.[37]

Acetylcysteine was licensed for use in 1968 and is on the WHO's List of Essential Medicines, the most effective and safe medicines needed in a health system. Intravenous and oral formulations of acetylcysteine are available for the treatment of paracetamol (acetaminophen) overdose.

NAC increases the levels of antioxidant and reduces glutathione at higher doses. Therefore, NAC has a potential to improve insulin receptor activity in human erythrocytes and improve insulin secretion in response to glucose.[38] Improvement in insulin receptor activity in hyperinsulinemic subjects can lead to a secondary decline in the β-cell responsiveness to the oral glucose tolerance test (OGTT). Decreased levels of circulating insulin can lead to significant reduction in testosterone levels and free androgen index in women responding to the treatment.[38, 39] Administration of NAC has many advantages including prevention of endothelial damage resulting from oxidants in noninsulin-dependent adult diabetic subjects and biological effects such as, protection against focal ischemia, phospholipid metabolism inhibition, proinflammatory cytokine release, and protease activity.[39] Therefore, it is suggested that the above effects exerted by NAC at the ovarian level may be as beneficial as its insulin-enhancing effects in inducing ovulation. In the absence of effective treatment options for PCOS, establishment of data on new options like NAC as monotherapy or supportive therapy may provide valuable information. No systematic reviews have assessed the effectiveness of NAC in PCOS.

The first clinical trial to investigate the metabolic effects of NAC was published in 1998. It identified a correlation between raised vascular cell adhesion molecule 1 (VCAM-1) plasma concentrations and reduced glutathione levels in untreated non-insulin dependent diabetes patients. It was theorized that oxidative stress contributes to the upregulation of VCAM-1 expression. With that in mind, supplementation with NAC was found to reduce its expression and, therefore, offer protection against diabetes-related endothelial damage.[40]

PCOS women have upregulated expression of VCAM-1, which shows positive correlation with elevated testosterone levels. Interventions like NAC that reduce VCAM-1 levels may consequentially reduce incidence of PCOS aggravation.[41]

In 2002, Fulghesu et al. conducted a study which studied improvements in insulin sensitivity and androgen levels with NAC supplementation. Reductions in triglyceride, total cholesterol, and low-density lipoprotein cholesterol levels were also observed. Most notably, this study highlighted the fact that NAC was well tolerated, producing little to no adverse effect.[38]

The meta-analysis from studies since 2002 suggests that NAC supplementation is worth considering for patients with PCOS. Whereas, it also suggests that metformin may be a superior treatment.[42]

A 2014 study raised concern suggesting that coadministration of NAC with metformin negates some of the benefits found when either is given alone. Serum levels of luteinizing hormone, testosterone, cholesterol, and triglycerides did not drop in the experimental group receiving both, whereas these parameters did improve when either NAC or metformin was administered alone. As a result of these findings, the authors suggest that combining NAC and metformin may not be useful for patients who are undergoing ovulation induction.[43]

Divyesh Thakker et al. in their systematic review, "N-acetylcysteine for Polycystic Ovary Syndrome: A Systematic Review and Meta-Analysis of Randomized Controlled Clinical Trials" published in the "Obstetrics and Gynecology International" (2015; 2015: 817849), reviewed the benefits and harms of N-acetylcysteine (NAC) in women with polycystic ovary syndrome (PCOS).

The review was conducted to assess clinical benefits and harms of NAC among women with PCOS. A total of eight randomized controlled trials with 910 women concluded that NAC significantly improved rates of live births and spontaneous ovulation compared to placebo in women with PCOS. However, they found no evidence of effects of NAC on improving menstrual regularity, acne, hirsutism, BMI, fasting insulin, fasting glucose, or HOMA-IR. NAC was not found superior to metformin for improving pregnancy rate, spontaneous ovulations, and in menstrual cycle regularity. But metformin improved the BMI, total testosterone, insulin level, and lipid levels compared to NAC. The side effect profiles were mild to moderate with no serious adverse drug events reported. Minor side effects were not reported in detail. All the studies were of short duration (three months) and long-term data on the comparative effects of NAC are lacking for important clinical outcomes such as resumption of menstrual regularity.

It may not be wrong to conclude that NAC certainly appears beneficial for PCOS patients, but metformin may be superior. Recommending these therapies simultaneously is probably not indicated until more evidence is available to show how the two work together.

CHROMIUM PICOLINATE

Chromium (III) picolinate ($CrPic_3$) is a chemical compound sold as a nutritional supplement to treat type 2 diabetes and promote weight loss.[44] This bright-red coordination compound is derived from chromium (III) and picolinic acid. Chromium in small quantity is needed for glucose utilization by insulin in normal health, but deficiency is extremely rare and has only been observed in people receiving 100% total parenteral nutrition diets.[45] Chromium has been identified as regulating insulin by increasing the sensitivity of the insulin receptor.[46] As such, chromium (III) picolinate has been proposed as a treatment for type 2 diabetes, although its effectiveness remains controversial due to conflicting evidence from human trials.[47]

A study in 1989 suggested that chromium (III) picolinate may aid in weight loss and in gaining muscle mass which led to an increased usage of chromium (III) picolinate supplements, resulting in it being for a while the second most widely used supplement behind

calcium.[47] A 2013 Cochrane review was unable to find "reliable evidence to inform firm decisions" to support such claims. Research has generally shown that it improves insulin sensitivity by either prolonging its activity or upregulating the production of mRNA to produce more insulin receptors.

Amongst the transition metals, Cr^{3+} is the most controversial in terms of nutritional value and toxicity. This controversy centres on whether Cr^{3+} provides any nutritional benefits. Furthermore, this controversy is amplified by the fact that no Cr-containing biomolecules have had their structure characterized, nor has the mode of action been determined. The first experiment that led to the discovery of Cr^{3+} playing a role in glucose metabolism proposed that the biologically active form of the metal existed in a protein called *glucose tolerance factor*, however, new evidence suggests that it is simply an artifact obtained from isolation procedures.[47] The only accepted indicator of chromium deficiency is the reversal of symptoms that occurs when chromium (III) supplementation is administered to people on total parenteral nutrition.

There are claims that the picolinate form of chromium supplementation aids in reducing insulin resistance and improving glucose metabolism, particularly in type 2 diabetics, but reviews showed no association between chromium and glucose or insulin concentrations for non-diabetics, and inconclusive results for diabetics.[48, 49] The authors of the second review mentioned that chromium picolinate decreased HbA1c levels by 0.7% in type 2 diabetes patients. They further observed that poor quality studies produced larger positive outcomes than higher quality studies.[49, 50] Two reviews concluded that chromium (III) picolinate may be more effective at lowering blood glucose levels compared to other chromium-containing dietary supplements.[49, 51]

The US Food and Drug Administration approved a qualified health claim for chromium picolinate as a dietary supplement relating to insulin resistance and risk of type 2 diabetes. Any company wishing to make such a claim must use the exact wording: "One small study suggests that chromium picolinate may reduce the risk of insulin resistance, and therefore, possibly may decrease the incidence of type 2 diabetes. FDA concludes, however, that the existence of such a relationship between chromium picolinate and either insulin resistance or type 2 diabetes is highly uncertain." As part of the petition review process, the FDA rejected other claims for reducing abnormally elevated blood sugar, risk of cardiovascular disease, risk of retinopathy or risk of kidney disease.[52] In 2006, the FDA added that the "relationship between chromium (III) picolinate intake and insulin resistance is highly uncertain".

There are no significant clinical results relating chromium (III) picolinate as adequate treatment of type 2 DM. It may be as a result of the degree of glucose intolerance of patients participating in the clinical studies. It has been shown that Cr (III) influences only glucose intolerance and not the insulin levels.

EL-Gharib et al. in 2014 compared the effects of N-acetylcysteine along with chromium picolinate on 120 PCOS women. They randomized the patients in three groups to receive either CC with NAC or CC with chromium and CC alone. They found that the number of follicles (≥18 mm), mean endometrial thickness on the day of hCG administration and number of pregnancies were higher among PCOS cases given NAC+CC group than CrP+CC and CC alone cases. In the group receiving CC+NAC, no significant side effects were noticed and only one case of OHSS was observed. Their conclusion was that NAC is a safe and well-tolerated adjuvant to CC and it also improves follicular maturation and pregnancy rate in PCOS patients. In addition, chromium picolinate does not improve follicular maturation or pregnancy rate when added to CC in women with PCOS.[53]

VITAMIN D

Vitamin D plays a physiological role in reproduction including ovarian follicular development and luteinization via altering anti-Müllerian hormone (AMH) signalling, follicle-stimulating hormone sensitivity and progesterone production in human granulosa cells.[54] It also affects glucose homeostasis through manifold roles. The potential influences of vitamin D on glucose homeostasis include the presence of specific vitamin D receptor (VDR) in pancreatic β-cells and skeletal muscle, the expression of 1-α-hydroxylase enzyme which can catalyze the conversion of 25-hydroxyvitamin D [25(OH)D] to 1,25-dihydroxyvitamin D, and the presence of a vitamin D response element in the human insulin gene promoter.[55]

The phenotypic manifestation of PCOS is associated with various degrees of gonadotropic and metabolic abnormalities determined by the interaction of multiple genetic and environmental factors. The prevalence of vitamin D deficiency in women with PCOS is about 67–85%, with serum concentrations of 25(OH)D <20 ng/mL.[56] Although there is no significant difference in the 25(OH)D levels between PCOS and normal control women, high prevalence of vitamin D deficiency has been found to be associated with metabolic syndrome which may have great impact on public health.[57] Low 25(OH)D levels may exacerbate the symptoms of PCOS, including insulin resistance, ovulatory, menstrual irregularities, infertility, hyperandrogenism, obesity and elevate the risk of cardiovascular diseases. Many observational studies suggest a possible role of vitamin D in an inverse association between vitamin D status and metabolic disturbances in PCOS, but it is still hard to draw a definite conclusion in the causal relationship due to inconsistent findings from a recent meta-analysis report of a systematic review.[58]

Vitamin D supplementation can lower the abnormally elevated serum AMH levels and increase serum anti-inflammatory soluble receptor for advanced glycation end-products in vitamin D-deficient women with PCOS.[54] In particular, vitamin D and calcium supplementation in addition to metformin therapy in women with PCOS could result in the beneficial effects on menstrual regularity and ovulation.[59] However, Garg et al.[60] recently demonstrated that there was no significant beneficial effect on insulin kinetics and cardiovascular risk factors after supplementation of vitamin D, at a dose of 4,000 IU/day for six months, among women with PCOS treated with metformin. Due to small sample size and the relatively short duration of follow up in previous observational study and clinical trial, the effects of vitamin D supplementation in relieving the symptoms in women with PCOS remain inconclusive.[59,60] Therefore, further research with high quality randomized controlled trials is warranted to establish the impact of vitamin D supplementation on the management of PCOS.

Low 25(OH)D levels are found to be significantly correlated with insulin resistance in women with PCOS.[55] Thus, genes involved in vitamin D metabolism have been suggested as candidate genes for the susceptibility to PCOS. A few polymorphisms in the *VDR* gene, such as Cdx2, Taq1, Bsm1, Apa1, and Fok1, were reported to play an influential role on insulin secretion and sensitivity in PCOS women.[61] The *VDR* Fok1 polymorphism was found to have a protective effect on the risk of type 2 diabetes mellitus, while the Bsm1 had a precipitating effect on the risk of type 2 diabetes. Besides, the Apa1 polymorphism was reported to confer a reduced risk of vitamin D deficiency.[61]

In this issue, Dasgupta et al.[62] present findings of a study conducted in Hyderabad, to investigate the association pattern of four *VDR* polymorphisms (Cdx2, Fok1, Apa1 and Taq1) with PCOS among Indian women. They found significant difference in the genotype and allele frequency distributions of the Cdx2 polymorphism between the PCOS and control women. A significantly higher frequency of the heterozygous GA genotype as well as the A allele of Cdx2 polymorphism was observed in controls when compared to cases ($P <0.001$), indicating a protective role of this single nucleotide polymorphism (SNP) against PCOS phenotype. After the adjustment of the covariates of age and body mass index, the carriers of GA genotype and the A allele remains conferring protecting effect for PCOS. However, no other significant associations were observed between the other three *VDR* polymorphisms (Fok1, Apa1 and Taq1) and PCOS. They further examined the associations between *VDR* genotypes and some of the PCOS specific clinical/biochemical traits, and found that the Cdx2 genotypes were significantly associated with testosterone levels and the Fok1 polymorphism showed a significant association with the presence of infertility. Further, the two haplotypes composed of four polymorphisms, ACCA and ACTA, were also found to be significantly associated with PCOS.

Despite several polymorphisms in *VDR* gene have been implicated in PCOS, the results from both individual research and meta-analysis in PCOS patients were in considerable disagreement and, therefore, the role of these variants of the *VDR* gene in the pathogenesis of insulin resistance and PCOS remains debatable. The inconsistent findings may be due to different ethnic origin or evolutionary force, such as genetic drift or selection pressure, or even due to different techniques of genotyping assay. For example, significant associations of the variant of insulin receptor substrate *(IRS)-2* gene as well as the interaction of *IRS-1* and *IRS-2* genes with PCOS were observed in a Chinese population of Taiwan that was contradictory to the findings from the meta-analysis conducted in Caucasian and African American populations.[63] Due to the wide heterogeneity of symptoms and signs of PCOS, which may be predisposed by different genetic and environmental factors, it may not be easy to evaluate putative functional correlations between *VDR* SNPs and PCOS. In addition, there are many interlinking factors which may affect the individual phenotypic expression of women with PCOS. So far, the role of vitamin D polymorphisms on metabolic disturbances in women with PCOS remains inconclusive. Further investigations with large independent cohorts as well as with diverse ethnic populations are necessary to clarify, if the relationship between vitamin D and PCOS is ethnic-specific or with different thresholds under the interactions of other individual genotypes of women with PCOS.

MELATONIN

Melatonin is a biogenic amine found in animals and plants. In mammals, melatonin is produced by the pineal gland with increased secretion in darkness and decline on exposure to light. Melatonin plays role in the sleep mood regulation and reproduction. Melatonin is also an effective antioxidant.

PCOS is considered to be the most common endocrine disorder affecting women. Melatonin influences sex steroid production at different stages of ovarian follicular maturation. Its receptors have been demonstrated at multiple sites in the ovary and in intrafollicular fluid. It plays role as an antioxidant and free radical scavenger which protects follicles from oxidative stress, rescuing them from atresia, leading to complete follicular maturation and ovulation.

Serum melatonin levels are significantly raised with hyperandrogenemia in women with PCOS along with increased number of atretic follicles. In a study conducted by Jain et al; the mean melatonin level was observed to be significantly increased in patients (63.27 ±10.97 pg/mL) than in controls (32.51 ±7.55 pg/mL). Melatonin was found to be raised in all the cases of PCOS (above cut-off value of ≥45 pg/mL, p < 0.001). Total testosterone level was raised in around 72% of patients. Melatonin levels were found to be positively correlated with increased testosterone (p <0.001).[64]

Further studies are needed required to recognize definite role of melatonin in PCOS cases with disturbed hormonal milieu which could open up the possible therapeutic role of melatonin in treatment of patients suffering from PCOS.

GLUCOCORTICOIDS

Adrenal steroidogenesis is under the influence of the hypothalamic–pituitary–adrenal axis. Insulin and obesity-related signals may play a role in the regulation of enzymes involved in the steroidogenetic pathways, as well as in the regulation of the HPA axis. In PCOS, cortisol production rate is probably normal, although there may be excessive adrenal androgens in a few women. Cortisol metabolism and regeneration from inactive glucocorticoids may also be disrupted in PCOS, leading to an adrenal hyperandrogenic state. Finally, over activity of the HPA axis may be related to the high prevalence of psychopathological and eating disorders in women with PCOS, implying a maladaptation in the adaptive mechanisms to chronic stress exposure.

Some women with PCOS have elevated adrenal androgen levels, although their contribution to ovulatory dysfunction appears modest.[65] Glucocorticoids suppress adrenal androgen secretion and thus have legitimate use in patients with classic congenital adrenal hyperplasia, where they can help prevent and manage hirsutism and allow ovulatory cycles. In non-classic congenital adrenal hyperplasia and functional adrenal androgen excess (a minority of PCOS patients), their role is more limited.[66] Adrenal androgens suppression can result in minor improvement of hirsutism. A trial of CPA versus hydrocortisone in patients with late-onset congenital adrenal hyperplasia showed a greater decrease in hirsutism scores with 1 year of CPA compared with hydrocortisone (54% vs 26%). These results occurred despite a greater reduction of androgens with glucocorticoids, highlighting the importance of peripheral receptivity to androgens.[67] Overdosing can occur, leading to adrenal atrophy, weight gain, and decreased bone mineral density. Glucocorticoid (5–7.5 mg of prednisone once or twice daily) has been shown to improve hirsutism in women with congenital adrenal hyperplasia. However, its effect on hirsutism due to other causes is unclear.[68] Unless a woman with PCOS has marked adrenal androgen excess, prolonged use of glucocorticoids is not advised.

Prednisone and dexamethasone have been used to induce ovulation in some cases. Elnashar et al. demonstrated that induction of ovulation by adding dexamethasone (high dose, short course) to CC in CC-resistant PCOS with normal DHEAS is associated with no adverse antioestrogenic effect on the endometrium and higher ovulation and pregnancy rates in a significant number of patients.[69]

In PCOS patients with high adrenal androgen, low-dose dexamethasone (0.25–0.5 mg) at bedtime can be used.[70] In a study of 230 women with PCOS who failed to ovulate with 200 mg of CC for 5 days, addition of 2 mg of dexamethasone from days 5–14 is associated with a higher ovulation rate and cumulative pregnancy rate.[71] Enthusiasm for their use is dampened, however, by their potential adverse effects on insulin sensitivity; therefore, prolonged use should be discouraged.

With the hypothesis that adrenal androgens (AA) excess in the form of dehydroepiandrosterone sulfate (DHEAS) is the main mechanism in anovulation considering it affects over 50% of PCOS woman, Aziz et al. conducted a very unique prospective study. Since AA could be suppressed by glucocorticoids, they selected 36 PCOS women in the age group of 18–40 years with clinical/biochemical evidence of hyperandrogenism and treated them with dexamethasone 0.5 mg/day for four cycles. Before and during the treatment period, the levels of free and total testosterone, SHBG, DHEA, DHEAS, androstenidione, cortisol, LH and FSH were measured. All patients showed significant reduction in all androgens (40–60%), a 24% increase in SHBG and no change in the LH/FSH. There was a mean increase of over 4 kg body weight at the end of therapy. Significantly 50% of the patients remained anovulatory and of the remaining patients; 28% had one ovulation, 14% had two and 8% had three ovulatory cycles. Data from this prospective study do not suggest treatment with glucocorticoids regardless of the basal DHEAS levels. It also had side effects mainly increase in the body weight. It may be concluded that although AA may be an important risk factor for PCOS, they play a limited role in ovulation.[72]

GROWTH HORMONE

Growth hormone (somatotropin or human growth hormone [hGH or HGH] in its human form), is a peptide hormone that stimulates growth, cell reproduction, and cell regeneration in humans and other animals. It is a type of mitogen specific only to certain kinds of cells. Growth hormone is a 191-amino acid, single-chain polypeptide that is synthesized, stored and secreted by somatotropic cells within the anterior pituitary gland.

It is a stress hormone that causes rise in the concentration of glucose and free fatty acids. It also stimulates production of IGF-1.

A recombinant form of hGH called somatropin (INN) is used to treat children's growth disorders and adult growth hormone deficiency.

hGH, due to its role as anabolic agent, has been used by competitors in sports since 1982, and has been banned by the IOC and NCAA. The use of this drug for performance enhancement is not currently approved by the FDA.

Several efforts have been made to obtain governmental approval for use GH in raising livestock more efficiently. These uses have been controversial. In the United States, the cow-specific form of GH called bovine somatotropin is used for increasing milk production in dairy cows (FDA approved).

Given recent *in vitro* and *in vivo* evidence that insulin and growth hormone may have gonadotropin-augmenting effects, the putative endocrine role of serum growth hormone levels in women with PCOS has been investigated in several studies. There is no correlation between IGF-1 and growth hormone in women with PCOS. Hyposomatotropinism in obese PCOS women is an obesity-dependent event. Evidence suggests that growth hormone may play a role in the lean PCOS woman and the obesity dampens its effect.

Growth hormone strongly contributes to the insulin resistance and hyperandrogenism in PCOS. Patients with pituitary tumors secreting growth hormone, develop several features overlapping with PCOS, including insulin resistance and hyperandrogenism. GH and its downstream effector hormone, insulin-like growth factor-1 (IGF-1), are increased in lean women with PCOS. It may be hypothesized that the excess insulin resistance and hyperandrogenism in PCOS are stimulated by increased growth hormone activity through IGF-1. A novel GH receptor antagonist (GHa), which is being used to treat acromegaly, provides a unique probe to test this hypothesis. GH receptor blockade has been shown to decrease insulin resistance in acromegaly.

In their study[73] (Homburg et al., 1995), 30 women with PCOS were given adjuvant growth hormone or placebo during GnRHa/gonadotropin therapy. Other than a GH-induced increase in serum insulin and IFG-1 concentrations, there were no significant differences between the growth hormone and placebo groups in gonadotropin requirement to attain ovulation, serum estradiol concentrations, number of growing follicles induced, nor in ovulation or pregnancy rates. They concluded that although growth hormone kinetics are abnormal and growth hormone pituitary reserves are suppressed in women with PCOS receiving GnRHa, the addition of growth hormone to this treatment regimen does not bestow any potential clinical benefit.

These findings, however, do not rule out the possible involvement of growth hormone in the pathogenesis of women with PCOS, predominantly in those of normal weight with no insulin resistance and normal insulin levels and who have an increased pituitary secretion and relatively high concentrations of growth hormone.[74] Indeed, these lean women with PCOS were found to have a mean growth hormone pulse amplitude that was elevated by 30% in comparison with lean controls (Morales et al., 1996) when growth hormone was frequently sampled over a 24-hour period. It was previously proposed that the high ovarian androgen concentrations in non-insulin resistant women with PCOS may be induced by growth hormone in a similar mechanism to that of insulin.[75]

In a recent study, de Boer et al. found that the pooled GH levels were significantly lower in PCOS patients than controls, as was GH pulse amplitude. There is no difference in number of GH pulses between PCOS patients and controls. Although a wide overlap between patients and controls was present, the M-value was significantly lower in PCOS patients. IGF-1 (insulin like growth factor-1) and IGFBP-3 (IGF binding protein-3) levels were not different between the groups. There was no correlation between the M-value and pooled GH or IGF-1 and IGFBP-3 levels. They concluded that non-obese patients with PCOS have impaired GH secretion and some but not all have impaired insulin sensitivity. These findings indicate that these patients may also be at risk for cardiovascular diseases and/or diabetes mellitus.[76]

ALTERNATIVE MEDICINE AND PCOS

Absence of evidence is not evidence of absence. Alternative medicine is being commonly practiced for different health problems. Alternative medicines include many modalities, such as kinesiology, herbalism, homeopathy, reflexology, acupressure, acupuncture, and massage therapy. Acupuncture is the most common modality. The benefit of acupuncture for PCOS sufferers is in helping them regulate and manage their periods, help in weight loss and reducing headaches as well as improving patients' moods and outlooks. Needles are placed along the acupuncture meridians related to the reproductive system. This helps to stimulate the organs, improves their blood supply, normalizes the hormone levels, and promotes the proper functioning of the reproductive system. A few studies have been performed on women with PCOS receiving acupuncture. In 2000, a study was carried out at Sweden involving 24 women with PCOS receiving acupuncture for 2–3 months. By the end of the study, nine women (38%) had regular ovulation. However, those women with more severe PCOS cases, particularly those having high testosterone and insulin levels and were obese, did not find any benefit with the acupuncture treatment.[77] Recently, a randomized controlled trial proved the efficacy of electroacupuncture in treating women with PCOS.[78]

In conclusion, it is clear that PCOS is an enigma. Its underlying pathophysiology is not fully understood. The treatments, so far, have been directed at the symptoms but not at the syndrome itself. Extensive efforts should be made to fully investigate the syndrome in order to make therapy more successful and to delay the serious long-term effects of the disease on patients' health.

REFERENCES

1. ESHRE/ASRM. Revised 2003 consensus on diagnostic criteria and long-term health risks related to polycystic ovary syndrome (PCOS). Hum Reprod 2004; 19: 41–47 [PubMed]
2. Azziz R, Carmina E, Dewailly D, Diamanti-Kandarakis E, Escobar-Morreale HF, Futterweit W, et al. (2006) Positions statement: criteria for defining polycystic ovary syndrome as a predominantly hyperandrogenic syndrome: an Androgen Excess Society guideline. J Clin Endocrinol Metab 91: 4237–4245 [PubMed]
3. Apridonidze T, Essah PA, Iuorno MJ, Nestler JE (2005) Prevalence and characteristics of the metabolic syndrome in women with polycystic ovary syndrome. J Clin Endocrinol Metab 90: 1929–1935 [PubMed]
4. Lisa J Moran, et.al. Endocrinol Metab Clin N Am 40 (2011) 895–906.
5. Franks S, et.al. Hum Reprod Update 2008; 14:367–78.
6. William Hurd et. al. Fertil Steril, Vol 96, Oct 2011).
7. Lifestyle changes in women with PCOS (Cochrane Review 2011) Hum. Reprod. (2008) 23 (3):462–477.
8. Bruner B, Chad K, Chizen D. Effects of exercise and nutritional counseling in women with polycystic ovary syndrome. Appl Physiol Nutr Metab. 2006;31(4):384–391. [PubMed]
9. Escobar-Morreale HF, Botella-Carretero JI, Alvarez-Blasco F, Sancho J, San Millán JL. The polycystic ovary syndrome associated with morbid obesity may resolve after weight loss induced by bariatric surgery. J Clin Endocrinol Metab. 2005;90(12):6364–6369. [PubMed]
10. Barbieri RL, Makris A, Randall RW, Daniels G, Kistner RW, Ryan KJ (1986) Insulin stimulates androgen accumulation in incubations of ovarian stroma obtained from women with hyperandrogenism. J Clin Endocrinol Metab 62: 904–910 [PubMed].
11. Nestler JE, Powers LP, Matt DW, Steingold KA, Plymate SR, Rittmaster RS, et al. (1991) A direct effect of hyperinsulinemia on serum sex hormone-binding globulin levels in obese women with polycystic ovary syndrome. J Clin Endocrinol Metab 72: 83–89 [PubMed]
12. Dunaif A, Graf M, Mandeli J, Laumas V, Dobrjansky A. (1987) Characterization of groups of hyperandrogenic women with acanthosis nigricans, impaired glucose tolerance, and/or hyperinsulinemia. J Clin Endocrinol Metab 65: 499–507 [PubMed]
13. Chang RJ, Laufer LR, Meldrum DR, DeFazio J, Lu JK, Vale WW, et al. (1983) Steroid secretion in polycystic ovarian disease after ovarian suppression by a long-acting gonadotropin-releasing hormone agonist. J Clin Endocrinol Metab 56:897–903 [PubMed]
14. DeUgarte CM, Bartolucci AA, Azziz R. (2005) Prevalence of insulin resistance in the polycystic ovary syndrome using the homeostasis model assessment. FertilSteril 83: 1454–1460 [PubMed]
15. Holte J, Bergh T, Berne C, Wide L, Lithell H. (1995) Restored insulin sensitivity but persistently increased early insulin secretion

after weight loss in obese women with polycystic ovary syndrome. J Clin Endocrinol Metab 80: 2586–2593 [PubMed]

16. Legro RS, Castracane VD, Kauffman RP. (2004) Detecting insulin resistance in polycystic ovary syndrome: purposes and pitfalls. Obstet Gynecol Surv 59:141–154 [PubMed]

17. Diamanti-Kandarakis E, Christakou CD, Kandaraki E, Economou FN. (2010) Metformin: an old medication of new fashion: evolving new molecular mechanisms and clinical implications in polycystic ovary syndrome. Eur J Endocrinol 162:193–212 [PubMed]

18. Nestler JE (2008) Metformin for the treatment of the polycystic ovary syndrome. N Engl J Med 358:47–54 [PubMed]

19. Ting RZ, Szeto CC, Chan MH, Ma KK, Chow KM (2006) Risk factors of vitamin B(12) deficiency in patients receiving metformin. Arch Intern Med 166:1975–1979 [PubMed]

20. Velazquez EM, Mendoza S, Hamer T, Sosa F, Glueck CJ (1994) Metformin therapy in polycystic ovary syndrome reduces hyperinsulinemia, insulin resistance, hyperandrogenemia, and systolic blood pressure, while facilitating normal menses and pregnancy. Metabolism 43:647–654 [PubMed]

21. Dunaif A, Scott D, Finegood D, Quintana B, Whitcomb R (1996) The insulin-sensitizing agent troglitazone improves metabolic and reproductive abnormalities in the polycystic ovary syndrome. J Clin Endocrinol Metab 81:3299–3306 [PubMed]

22. Nieuwenhuis-Ruifrok AE, Kuchenbecker WK, Hoek A, Middleton P, Norman RJ (2009) Insulin sensitizing drugs for weight loss in women of reproductive age who are overweight or obese: systematic review and meta-analysis. Hum Reprod Update 15:57–68 [PubMed]

23. Mansfield R, Galea R, Brincat M, Hole D, Mason H (2003) Metformin has direct effects on human ovarian steroidogenesis. FertilSteril 79:956–962 [PubMed]

24. Lord JM, Flight IH, Norman RJ (2003) Insulin-sensitising drugs (metformin, troglitazone, rosiglitazone, pioglitazone, D-chiro-inositol) for polycystic ovary syndrome. Cochrane Database Syst Rev 3: CD003053. [PubMed]

25. Palomba S, Pasquali R, Orio F, Jr, Nestler JE (2009) Clomiphene citrate, metformin or both as first-step approach in treating anovulatory infertility in patients with polycystic ovary syndrome (PCOS): a systematic review of head-to-head randomized controlled studies and meta-analysis. Clin Endocrinol (Oxf) 70:311–321 [PubMed]

26. Tso LO, Costello MF, Albuquerque LE, Andriolo RB, Freitas V (2009) Metformin treatment before and during IVF or ICSI in women with polycystic ovary syndrome. Cochrane Database Syst Rev 2: CD006105. [PubMed]

27. Doldi N, Persico P, Di Sebastiano F, Marsiglio E, Ferrari A (2006) Gonadotropin-releasing hormone antagonist and metformin for treatment of polycystic ovary syndrome patients undergoing in vitro fertilization-embryo transfer. Gynecol Endocrinol 22:235–238 [PubMed]

28. Tang T, Lord JM, Norman RJ, Yasmin E, Balen AH Insulin-sensitising drugs (metformin, rosiglitazone, pioglitazone, D-chiro-inositol) for women with polycystic ovary syndrome, oligo amenorrhoea and subfertility. Cochrane Database Syst Rev. 2012 May 16; (5):CD003053.)

29. Attia GR, Rainey WE, Carr BR (2001) Metformin directly inhibits androgen production in human thecal cells. Fertil Steril 76:517–524 [PubMed]

30. Bailey CJ, Turner RC (1996) Metformin. N Engl J Med 334:574–579 [PubMed]

31. Harborne L, Fleming R, Lyall H, Sattar N, Norman J (2003) Metformin or antiandrogen in the treatment of hirsutism in polycystic ovary syndrome. J Clin Endocrinol Metab 88: 4116–4123 [PubMed]

32. Nestler JE, Jakubowicz DJ (1997) Lean women with polycystic ovary syndrome respond to insulin reduction with decreases in ovarian P450c17 alpha activity and serum androgens. J Clin Endocrinol Metab 82: 4075–4079 [PubMed]

33. Pasquali R, Gambineri A, Biscotti D, Vicennati V, Gagliardi L, Colitta D, et al. (2000) Effect of long-term treatment with metformin added to hypocaloric diet on body composition, fat distribution, and androgen and insulin levels in abdominally obese women with and without the polycystic ovary syndrome. J Clin Endocrinol Metab 85:2767–2774 [PubMed]

34. Bizzarri M, Fuso A, Dinicola S, Cucina A, Bevilacqua A. Pharmacodynamics and pharmacokinetics of inositol(s) in health and disease. Expert Opinion on Drug Metabolism and Toxicology 2016. 12 1181–1196. (10.1080/17425255.2016.1206887) [PubMed]

35. Vittorio Unfer, Fabio Facchinetti, Beatrice Orrù, Barbara Giordani,[3] and John Nestler[4] Myo-

inositol effects in women with PCOS: a meta-analysis of randomized controlled trialsInt J Endocrinol. 2016; 2016: 9537632. Endocr Connect. 2017 Nov; 6(8): 647–658.

36. Pedro-Antonio Regidor[1], and Adolf Eduard Schindler[2] Myoinositol as a Safe and Alternative Approach in the Treatment of Infertile PCOS Women: A German Observational Study: Int J Endocrinol. 2016; 2016: 9537632.

37. Acetylcysteine, The American Society of Health System Pharmacicts: Archived from the original on 23 September 2015. Retrieved 22 august 2015.

38. Fulghesu AM, Ciampelli M, Muzj G, et al. N-acetyl-cysteine treatment improves insulin sensitivity in women with polycystic ovary syndrome. *Fertility and Sterility*. 2002;77(6):1128–1135. doi: 10.1016/s0015-0282(02)03133-3. [PubMed] [Cross Ref]

39. Elnashar A, Fahmy M, Mansour A, Ibrahim K N-acetyl cysteine vs. metformin in treatment of clomiphene citrate-resistant polycystic ovary syndrome: a prospective randomized controlled study. *Fertility and Sterility*. 2007;88(2):406–409. doi: 10.1016/j.fertnstert.2006.11.173. [PubMed] [Cross Ref]

40. De Mattia G, Bravi MC, Laurenti O, et al. Reduction of oxidative stress by oral N-acetyl-L-cysteine treatment decreases plasma soluble vascular cell adhesion molecule-1 concentrations in non-obese, non-dyslipidaemic, normotensive, patients with non-insulin-dependent diabetes. *Diabetologia*. 1998;41(11):1392–1396.

41. Solano ME, Sander VA, Ho H, Motta AB, Arck PC. Systemic inflammation, cellular influx and up-regulation of ovarian VCAM-1 expression in a mouse model of polycystic ovary syndrome (PCOS). *J Reprod Immunol*. 2011;92(1-2):33–44.

42. Fulghesu AM, Ciampelli M, Muzj G, et al. N-acetyl-cysteine treatment improves insulin sensitivity in women with polycystic ovary syndrome. *Fertil Steril*. 2002; 77(6):1128–1135.

43. Cheraghi E, Soleimani Mehranjani M, Shariatzadeh MA, Nasr Esfahni MH, Ebrahimi Z. Co-administration of metformin and N-acetyl cysteine fails to improve clinical manifestations in PCOS individual undergoing ICSI. *Int J FertilSteril*. 2014;8(2):119-128.

44. Preuss, HG; Echard, B; Perricone, NV; Bagchi, D; Yasmin, T; Stohs, SJ (2008). "Comparing metabolic effects of six different commercial trivalent chromium compounds". Journal of Inorganic Biochemistry. 102 (11): 1986–1990.

doi:10.1016/j.jinorgbio.2008.07.012. PMID 18774175

45. Review of Chromium Archived February 7, 2012, at the Wayback Machine. Expert Group on Vitamins and Minerals Review of Chromium, 12 August 2002.

46. Stearns DM (2000). "Is chromium a trace essential metal?". BioFactors. 11 (3): 149–62. doi:10.1002/biof.5520110301. PMID 10875302.

47. Vincent, John (2010). "Chromium: celebrating 50 years as an essential element?". Dalton Transactions. Royal Society of Chemistry. 39: 3787–3794. doi:10.1039/B920480F. PMID 20372701. Retrieved 20 March 2015.

48. Althuis MD, Jordan NE, Ludington EA, Wittes JT (1 July 2002). "Glucose and insulin responses to dietary chromium supplements: a meta-analysis". American Journal of Clinical Nutrition. 76 (1): 148–155. PMID 12081828.

49. Balk EM, Tatsioni A, Lichtenstein AH, Lau J, Pittas AG (2007). "Effect of chromium supplementation on glucose metabolism and lipids: a systematic review of randomized controlled trials". Diabetes Care. 30 (8): 2154–2163. doi:10.2337/dc06-0996. PMID 17519436.

50. Suksomboon, N.; Poolsup, N.; Yuwanakom, A. (2014). "Systematic review and meta-analysis of the efficacy and safety of chromium supplementation in diabetes". Journal of Clinical Pharmacy and Therapeutics. John Wiley and Sons. 39 (3): 292–306. doi:10.1111/jcpt.12147. Retrieved 30 March 2015.

51. Broadhurst CL, Domenico P (December 2006). "Clinical studies on chromium picolinate supplementation in diabetes mellitus—a review". Diabetes Technol. Ther. 8 (6): 677–87. doi:10.1089/dia.2006.8.677. PMID 17109600.

52. Qualified Health Claims: Letter of Enforcement Discretion–Chromium Picolinate and Insulin Resistance(Docket No. 2004Q-0144) (2005) US Food and Drug Administration.

53. EL-Gharib MN1 and Osman AM2 Medicine, Tanta University, Tanta, Egypt Research Article **www.enlivenarchive.org** Enliven: Gynecology and Obstetrics: N-Acetyl Cysteine, Chromium Picolinate: Adjuvant to Clomiphene Therapy of PCOS.

54. Irani M, Merhi Z. Role of vitamin D in ovarian physiology and its implication in reproduction: a systematic review. FertilSteril. 2014;102:460-8.e3. [PubMed]

55. Alvarez JA, Ashraf A. Role of vitamin D in insulin secretion and insulin sensitivity for glucose homeostasis. Int J Endocrinol 2010. 2010:ID351385. [PubMed]

56. Thomson RL, Spedding S, Buckley JD. Vitamin D in the aetiology and management of polycystic ovary syndrome. Clin Endocrinol (Oxf) 2012;77:343–50. [PubMed]

57. Moini A, Shirzad N, Ahmadzadeh M, Hosseini R, Hosseini L, Sadatmahalleh SJ. Comparison of 25-hydroxyvitamin D and calcium levels between polycystic ovarian syndrome and normal women. Int J FertilSteril. 2015;9:1–8. [PMC free article] [PubMed]

58. Krul-Poel YH, Snackey C, Louwers Y, Lips P, Lambalk CB, Laven JS, et al. The role of vitamin D in metabolic disturbances in polycystic ovary syndrome: a systematic review. Eur J Endocrinol. 2013;169:853–65. [PubMed]

59. Rashidi B, Haghollahi F, Shariat M, Zayerii F. The effects of calcium-vitamin D and metformin on polycystic ovary syndrome: a pilot study. Taiwan J Obstet Gynecol. 2009;48:142–7. [PubMed]

60. Garg G, Kachhawa G, Ramot R, Khadgawat R, Tandon N, Sreenivas V, et al. Effect of vitamin D supplementation on insulin kinetics and cardio-vascular risk factors in polycystic ovarian syndrome: a pilot study. Endocr Connect. 2015; 4:108–16. [PubMed]

61. Al-Daghri NM, Al-Attas OS, Alkharfy KM, Khan N, Mohammed AK, Vinodson B, et al. Association of VDR-gene variants with factors related to the metabolic syndrome, type 2 diabetes and vitamin D deficiency. Gene. 2014;542:129–33. [PubMed]

62. Dasgupta S, Dutta J, Annameneni S, Kudugunti N, Mohan Reddy B. Association of vitamin D receptor gene polymorphisms with polycystic ovary syndrome among Indian women. Indian J Med Res. 2015;142:276–85. [PMC free article] [PubMed]

63. Lin MW, Huang MF, Wu MH. Association of Gly972Arg variant of insulin receptor subtrate-1 and Gly1057Asp variant of insulin receptor subtrate-2 with polycystic ovary syndrome in the Chinese population. J Ovarian Res. 2014;7:92. [PMC free article] [PubMed]

64. Jain P[1], Jain M[1], Haldar C[2], Singh TB[3], Jain S[1].Melatonin and its correlation with testosterone in polycystic ovarian syndrome. J Hum Reprod Sci. 2013 Oct;6(4):253–8. doi: 10.4103/0974–1208.126295.

65. Azziz R, Black V, Hines GA, Fox LM, Boots LR. Adrenal androgen excess in the polycystic ovary syndrome: sensitivity and responsivity of the hypothalamic-pituitary-adrenal axis. J Clin Endocrinol Metab. 1998;83(7):2317–2323. [PubMed]

66. Sahin Y, Dilber S, Kelestimur F. Comparison of Diane 35 and Diane 35 plus finasteride in the treatment of hirsutism. Fertil Steril. 2001; 75(3):496–500. [PubMed]

67. Spritzer P, Billaud L, Thalabard JC, et al. Cyproterone acetate versus hydrocortisone treatment in late-onset adrenal hyperplasia. J Clin Endocrinol Metab. 1990;70(3):642–646. [PubMed]

68. Lumachi F, Rondinone R. Use of cyproterone acetate, finasteride, and spironolactone to treat idiopathic hirsutism. Fertil Steril. 2003;79(4):942–946. [PubMed]

69. Elnashar A, Abdelmageed E, Fayed M, Sharaf M. Clomiphene citrate and dexamethazone in treatment of clomiphene citrate-resistant polycystic ovary syndrome: a prospective placebo-controlled study. Hum Reprod. 2006;21(7):1805–1808. [PubMed]

70. Nugent D, Vandekerckhove P, Hughes E, Arnot M, Lilford R. Gonadotrophin therapy for ovulation induction in subfertility associated with polycystic ovary syndrome. Cochrane Database Syst Rev. 2000;(4):CD000410. doi: 10.1002/14651858.CD000410. [PubMed]

71. Parsanezhad ME, Alborzi S, Motazedian S, Omrani G. Use of dexamethasone and clomi-phene citrate in the treatment of clomiphene citrate-resistant patients with polycystic ovary syndrome and normal dehydroepiandrosterone sulfate levels: a prospective, double-blind, placebo-controlled trial. Fertil Steril. 2002; 78(5):1001–1004. [PubMed]

72. Azziz R[1], Black VY, Knochenhauer ES, Hines GA, Boots LR. Ovulation after glucocorticoid suppression of adrenal androgens in the polycystic ovary syndrome is not predicted by the basal dehydroepiandrosterone sulfate level. J Clin Endocrinol Metab. 1999 Mar;84(3):946–50.

73. Homburg, R., Levy, T. and Ben-Rafael, Z. (1995) Adjuvant growth hormone for induction of ovulation with gonadotrophin-releasing hormone agonist and gonadotrophins in polycystic ovary syndrome: a randomised, double blind, placebo controlled trial. *Hum. Reprod.*, 10, 2550–2553

74. Prelevic, G.M., Wurzburger, M.I., Balint-Peric, L. and Ginsburg, J. (1992) Twenty-four hour serum growth hormone, insulin, C-peptide and blood glucose profiles and serum insulin-like growth factor-1 concentrations in women with polycystic ovaries. *Horm. Res.*, 37, 125–131.

75. Homburg, R., Levy, T., Orvieto, R. and Ben-Rafael, Z. (1996) The effect of growth hormone administration on serum concentrations of insulin-like growth factor-1, IGF binding protein-1 and insulin in women with polycystic ovary syndrome. *Israel J. Obstet. Gynecol.*, 7, 1–3.

76. de Boer JA[1], Lambalk CB, Hendriks HH, van Aken C, van der Veen EA, Schoemaker J. Growth hormone secretion is impaired but not related to insulin sensitivity in non-obese patients with polycystic ovary syndrome. Hum Reprod. 2004 Mar;19(3):504-9. Epub 2004 Jan 29.

77. Stener-Victorin E, Waldenström U, Tägnfors U, Lundeberg T, Lindstedt G, Janson PO. Effects of electro-acupuncture on anovulation in women with polycystic ovary syndrome. Acta Obstet Gynecol Scand. 2000;79(3):180–188. [PubMed]

78. Jedel E, Labrie F, Odén A, et al. Impact of electro-acupuncture and exercise on hyperandrogenism and oligo/amenorrhoea in women with polycystic ovary syndrome: a randomized controlled trial. Am J Physiol Endocrinol Metab. 2010 Oct 13; Epub ahead of print. [PubMed]

15

Ovulation Induction in PCOS: Clomiphene Citrate

Sukesh Kumar Kathpalia, Amey Chugh

There are many challenges in the management of polycystic ovarian syndrome (PCOS); inability to conceive is the biggest challenge[1] for both; the doctor and the patient. Anovulation or infrequent ovulation is the commonest cause of infertility in PCOS.[2] Many times PCOS is discovered when the couple is being investigated for infertility. Before embarking on ovulation induction; it is necessary to exclude other causes as more than one factor may be associated with anovulation. Clomiphene citrate (CC) is the most frequently used medication for induction of ovulation and is in clinical use for more than five decades.[3]

CC belongs to the group of medicines called selective estrogen receptor modulator (SERM); its chemical structure is similar to estrogen and has both antiestrogenic and estrogenic actions.[4] It binds to the estrogen receptors in hypothalamus and causes release of GnRH which in turn stimulates anterior pituitary gland to secrete follicle stimulating hormone (FSH) that acts on the ovaries and initiates the cycle of ovulation. CC inhibits the negative feedback of estrogen on hypothalamus thereby leading to upregulation of hypothalamic–pituitary–ovarian (HPO) axis.

The medicine is marketed by different names with the strength of 50 mg per tablet. Starting of medicine should be at the proper time and best results are obtained, if started from second or third day of the menstrual cycle and the process of ovulation monitored by transvaginal sonography (TVS), serum estradiol levels, LH surge or cervical mucous studies. Serum progesterone may be measured during midluteal phase and indicate ovulation if levels are more than 10 ng/mL. Many patients of PCOS have amenorrhea and CC should be started after withdrawal bleed with progestogens; first day of withdrawal bleed to be taken as first day of menstruation. Usual starting dose is 50 mg per day for five days; the medicine can be taken anytime of the day but preferably should be taken at the same time everyday. The drug may be repeated in incremental doses of 50 mg increase every month, the maximum recommended dose is 150 mg and should not be given for more than six cycles. Consumption of CC for more than 12 cycles has been associated with increased incidence of epithelial ovarian cancer.[5]

Clomiphene may administered alone[6] or with metformin[7] in cases of PCOS, combination of the two gives better results especially in obese cases.[8,9] But reliable studies and protocols of CC and metformin are not available.[1,10,11] CC may be combined with gonadotropins in cases where ovulation and or conception do not occur even after prolonged use of CC for 12 months.[12,13] Aromatase inhibitors Letrozole; too is an effective ovulation inducing drug.[14,15] Most of the women on CC will ovulate 8 to 10 days after the last dose. Most of the patients respond and ovulate in first two to three cycles. The chances of conception are reduced thereafter due to its anti-estrogenic actions. But this can vary; some of them may ovulate and conceive even two to three weeks after the last CC tablet was consumed. There is a mismatch between ovulation and conception rate; the reason of that has been thought to be antiestrogenic properties of CC.

If the outcome after six months is not favorable, the modality of ovulation should be changed. Incidence of congenital malformations in babies conceived after CC is not higher than in babies conceived after natural ovulation. CC is a relatively safe drug; the two common side effects of concern are multiple pregnancies and multiple births due to multiple ovulation. Ovarian hyperstimulation syndrome (OHSS)[16] which is not so common but is dangerous. Other minor side effects being:

- Nausea and vomiting
- Flushing and hot flashes due to its anti-estrogenic actions
- Cervical mucus becomes thick due to its antiestrogenic action on cervical mucus glands; which may interfere with sperm penetration. Intrauterine insemination will circumvent this problem.
- Mood changes, irritability and depression
- Headache and blurred vision
- Breast tenderness
- Pain abdomen or pelvic pain which may be due to enlarged ovaries.

Most of the minor side effects are manageable and rarely require any intervention. Serious side effects are very rare. Some patients may be allergic to CC. Severity of the side effects is dose dependent, and these side effects disappear dramatically after stopping CC. The contraindications to prescribing CC are:

- Abnormal vaginal bleeding
- Liver disease
- Severe thyroid and adrenal disorders
- Pituitary tumor

Final Message

1. Clomiphene is the first line of treatment for anovulatory infertility in patients who are not obese. It is cheap, easy to administer, has minimum side effects and monitoring is easy.
2. Patients who are obese (BMI >30 kg/m^2), clomiphene with metformin gives better results.
3. Poor responders should be shifted to other medicines for ovulation induction. It is a difficult decision especially in those cases who ovulate but do not conceive.

REFERENCES

1. Aqueela A, Alwan Y, Farooq MU. Metformin-clomiphene citrate vs clomiphene citrate alone: Polycystic ovarian syndrome. J Hum Reprod Sci 2013;6(1):15–18.
2. Costello MF. Theme: Polycystic ovary syndrome - a management update. Aust Fam Physician 2005;34:127–33.
3. Pritts E. Letrozole for ovulation induction and controlled ovarian Hyperstimulation. Current options. Obstetrics & Gynecology 2010;22:289–94.
4. Shelly W, et al. Selective estrogen receptor modulators: An update on recent clinical findings. Obstetrical & Gynecological Survey 2008; 63:163–81.
5. Rossing M, Daling J, Weiss N. Ovarian tumors in a cohort of infertile women. New England Journal of Medicine 1994;331:1165–74.
6. Zain MM, Jamaluddin R, Ibrahim A, Norman RJ. Comparison of clomiphene citrate, metformin, or the combination of both for first-line ovulation induction, achievement of pregnancy, and live birth in Asian women with polycystic ovary syndrome: A randomized controlled trial. Fertil Steril 2009;91:514–21.
7. Neveu N, Granger L, St-Michel P, Lavoie HB. Comparison of clomiphene citrate, metformin, or the combination of both for first-line ovulation induction and achievement of pregnancy in 154 women with polycystic ovary syndrome. Fertil Steril 2007;87:113–20.
8. Paloma S, et al. Evidence-bases and potential benefits of metformin in the polycystic ovary syndrome: a comprehensive review. Endocrine Reviews 2009;30(1):1–50.
9. Morley LC, et al. Insulin sensitizing drugs (metformin, rosiglitazone, pioglitazone, D-chiro-inositol) for women with polycystic ovary syndrome, oligomenorrhoea and subfertility. Cochrane Database Syst Rev 2017; 11.

10. Hoeger KM, et al. A randomized, 48 weeks, placebo-controlled trial of intensive life style modification and/or metformin therapy in overweight women with polycystic ovary syndrome: a pilot study. Fertility & Sterility. 2004;82(2):421–9.

11. Robert J, Helena H, Teede J. Long versus short course treatment with metformin and clomiphene citrate for ovulation induction in women with PCOS. Human Reproduction Update. 2013;19(1):2–11.

12. Abu Hashim, Bazeed HM, I Abd Elaal, Minimal stimulation or clomiphene citrate as first-line therapy in women polycystic ovary syndrome: a randomized controlled trial. Gynecol Endrocrinol 2012;28(2):87–90.

13. Mukherjee S, Sharma S, Chakravarty BN. Comparative evaluation of pregnancy outcome in gonadotrophin-clomiphene combination vs clomiphene alone in polycystic ovarian syndrome and unexplained infertility-A prospective clinical trial. J Hum Reprod Sci 2010; 3(2):80–84.

14. Mitwally M, Casper R. Use of an aromatase inhibitor for induction of ovulation in patients with an inadequate response to clomiphene citrate. Fertility & Sterility 2001;75:305–09.

15. Elizur S, Tuland T. Drugs in infertility and fetal safety. Fertility & Sterility. 2008;89:1595–1602.

16. Kafy S and Tulandi T. New advances in ovulation induction. Current opinion in Obstetrics and Gynecology 2009;21:465–73.

Ovulation Induction in PCOS: Gonadotropins

Chandrakant S Madkar, Rajendra Shitole

PCOS is a heterogeneous collection of signs and symptoms which form a spectrum of mild to severe disturbances of reproductive endocrine and metabolic function.[1] In fact, it represents the commonest cause of normo-gonadotropic anovulation accounting for 90% of WHO-II cohort.[2] It was actually described by Stein-Leventhal in women with hirsutism, amenorrhea, obesity and enlarged bilateral polycystic ovaries.[3] In 1960, it was popularly described as PCOS throughout the world.

Features of PCOS[4]

- 5–10% of women are in reproductive age.
- 30–40% of women with secondary amenorrhea.
- More than 70% women having anovulation leading to infertility.
- 30% women are obese.
- 90% women represent with hirsutism and regular menses.

Diagnostic Criteria

Different institutions like NIH (National Institute of Child Health), ESHRE/ASRM (European Society for Human Reproduction and Embryology/American Society for Reproductive Medicine), AEPCOS (Androgen Excess and PCOS Society) have given different diagnostic criteria. However, in practice, we are following ESHRE/ASRM criteria which are defined by Rotterdam consensus 2003.[5]

The criteria mentioned by them are as follows:
1. Oligo- and/or anovulation.
2. Hyperandrogenism (clinical and/or biochemical).
3. Polycystic ovaries with exclusion of other etiologies.

Radiological criteria to define PCOS are:[6]
1. Presence of 12 or more cysts of 2–9 mm
2. Ovarian volume equal to more than 12 cm
3. Bright echogenic stroma

As our topic is related with ovulation induction in PCOS with gonadotropins, the upcoming discussion will be focused on this topic. In about 30–40% of infertility patients, disturbance of ovulation is observed.

WHO has categorized anovulation in three groups:[7]
- Group I   Hypothalamic pituitary failure (hypogonadotropic hypogonadism)
- Group II   Hypothalamic pituitary dysfunction (normogonadotropic anovulation, e.g. PCOD)
- Group III Ovarian failure (hypergonadotropic hypogonadism)

GONADOTROPIN

Menstruation cycle is regulated by neuro-endocrinology control through HPO axis and gonadotropin is the middle step of this ladder. The gonadotropins (LH and FSH) are secreted by the anterior pituitary gonadotrophs which are basophilic cells under the influence of pulsatile GnRH stimulation. They are responsible for follicular selection, dominance, ovulation and functioning of corpus luteum. They also stimulate the synthesis of estrogen, progesterone and peptides in the ovaries. These exert negative feedback at hypothalamic pituitary level due to which there is decrease in gonadotropin secretions, which is responsible for single dominant follicle developing in a normal menstruation cycle. The increase in estradiol levels initiate the positive feedback effect on hypothalamus and pituitary which is responsible for pre-ovulatory gonadotropin surge.[4] The third gonadotropin hCG, i.e. human chorionic gonadotropin comes into action after fertilization, the function of which is to support pregnancy.

Structure of Gonadotropin

These are glycoprotein hormones which are composed of two non-covalently linked protein subunits, i.e. alpha and beta. They are attached to carbohydrate moieties. The alpha subunit is composed of 92 amino acids. Whereas, beta subunits are different and confer the unique biological and immuno-logical properties and receptors specificities of each of these glycoproteins. The subunits alone have no biological activity. It is the formation of hetero-dimer that provides the hormonal activity through attachment of the carbohydrate moieties. The extent of glycosylation and especially sylation, that conveys the spectrum of differences in charge, bioactivities, elimination and half-lives.

FSH

- It plays an important role in gametogenesis in both the partners, i.e male and female.
- In men, it is required for the establishment and maintenance of spermatogenesis.
- In women it stimulates the growth of ovarian follicle and fluctuations in each

secretion are involved in the selection of the ovulatory follicle.

- The beta subunit of FSH is composed of 111 amino acids.
- The multiple forms of FSH with variable compositions differ in their plasma half-life due to variation in their binding potential.
- The distribution of isoform types is under endocrine control and amount of sialic acid present is influenced mainly by estradiol (E2) levels. The higher the E2 levels, the less glycosylated FSH , the shorter the half-life but the greater receptor affinity.[4]

LH and hCG

- Although the alpha subunits of LH and hCG are identical to that of FSH, the beta subunits are different.
- LH has a beta subunit containing 121 amino acids that confer its specific biological action which is responsible for its interaction with LH receptors.
- These beta subunits of LH contain the same amino acids in sequence like hCG. But the hCG beta units contain additional 23 amino acids.
- The two hormones differ in composition of their carbohydrate moieties which in turn affect the bioactivity and half-life.
- The half-life of LH is 20 minutes and that of hCG is 24 hours.[4]

Indications for Gonadotropin

1. Hypothalamic pituitary insufficiency/dysfunction.
2. The failure of clomiphene/letrozole
3. The intolerable side effects to clomiphene and letrozole
4. Controlled ovarian hyperstimulation (COH in ART)
5. Premature luteinization of follicles
6. Unexplained infertility
7. PCOS

Prerequisite for the Patient to be Started on Gonadotropin[1]

1. Detailed counselling regarding need for treatment, monitoring required, its success rate alternative therapy cost and risk of multiple pregnancy and hyperstimulation.
2. Screening to rule out other factors which are responsible for the infertility.
3. Baseline transvaginal ultrasonography.
4. Day 2—LH, FSH and estradiol .
5. Rule out other endocrinopathies like-hyperprolactinemia and thyroid dysfunction.
6. Rule out ovarian tumors.

Contraindications for Gonadotropin[4]

1. Hypersensitivity
2. Tumors of hypothalamus and pituitary gland
3. Ovarian cyst
4. Abnormal uterine bleeding
5. Genital and breast cancer
6. Premature ovarian failure

Side Effects of Gonadotropin[4]

1. *Immunity system:* Mild erythema, rash and anaphylactic reaction
2. *Nervous system:* Headache
3. *Respiratory system:* Exacerbation of asthma
4. *Vascular system:* Thromboembolism
5. *GI system:* Nausea, vomiting, diarrhea and bloating
6. *Reproductive system:* Ovarian cyst, ovarian hyperstimulation syndrome and ovarian torsion
7. *Administration site:* Pain, redness, swelling, bruising and irritation

Production of Gonadotropin and Preparations Available

Human menopausal gonadotropin (HMG) was first extracted in 1953 from urine of menopausal woman. This contained FSH and LH in the ratio of 1:1. The first birth after gonadotropin simulation was reported by Alan Trounson in 1981.[7] Subsequently, FSH with LH separated by polyvalent antibodies and made commercially available in 1987. A highly purified FSH was obtained by removing LH by monoclonal antibodies. Finally, the recombinant technology was used for FSH preparation with absolutely no LH activity.

Gonadotropin Preparations

1. Human pituitary gonadotropin.
2. Human menopausal gonadotropin containing 75 international unit of FSH and LH.
3. Highly purified HMG containing 75 IU of FSH and LH but less than 5% of urine protein.
4. Purified urinary FSH-75 IU of FSH and less than 0.7 IU of LH.
5. Highly purified urinary FSH which contains 75 IU FSH and less than 0.001 IU of LH.
6. Recombinant FSH containing pure FSH and no LH.
7. Recombinant LH

Note: The introduction in 1996 of the first recombinant FSH followed by recombinant hCG and then LH brought about radical change in the quality standardization and availability of gonadotropin.

The following advantages of recombinant FSH brought about radical change in quality, standardization and availability of gonadotropins:

1. High purity
2. Specific activity
3. Unlimited supply with batch to batch consistency
4. Absolute monohormonal products
5. Less immune reactions
6. Subcutaneous self-administration
7. Ready to use pen devices
8. Superior quality control

Further research is going on the preparation of long-acting LH, and FSH.

Gonadotropin Therapy

The principle of ovulation induction with gonadotropin relies on the fact that initiation and maintenance of follicle growth is brought about by transient increase in the duration of FSH level above the threshold to recruit a limited number of developing follicle.[8]

Different types of protocols that are in use are as follows.

1. Step-up Protocols

There are two types of step-up protocols.
a. Low dose step-up protocol
b. Chronic low dose step-up protocol
- In these protocols, there is step-wise increase in FSH dose to determine the FSH threshold for follicular development.
- Starting dose of protocol is 37.5–75 IU.
- In the low dose step-up protocol, the selected dose of gonadotropin is given for a week and then assessed for follicular growth and estradiol levels. If it is not satisfactory, then the dose is increased by 75 IU.
- Once, the growth is seen, the same dose is maintained till follicular selection is achieved.[8–11]
- In chronic low dose step-up protocols, the initial selected dose is given for 14 days and then follicular growth is assessed. If growth is not satisfactory, then weekly increment of 37.5 IU are made till follicular growth is seen. And thereafter, the same dose is maintained till follicular selection. This regime is intended at reducing the risk of hyper-response to stimulation.

2. Step-down Protocols

- This protocol is designed to match the physiology of the normal cycle.
- An initial high loading dose of FSH is given which is intended to cross the FSH intended level by step-wise reduction in the dose following follicular development.

3. Sequential Step-up, Step-down Regime

- It is started like step up protocol but the dose is reduced by half when the follicle is 14 mm.
- This approach reduces the number lead follicles and is suitable for PCOS patients.[12]
- Sequential therapy is useful only in women who respond to clomiphene at least to some extent.
- While on treatment, strict monitoring is done by follicular study on ultrasonography and serum estradiol levels. And the ovulation can be triggered after follicle achieves 18–20 mm size with hCG injection.
- The endometrial thickness also should be monitored.

Complications of Gonadotropin Therapy

1. Multiple pregnancy is found in about 10–40% patients. Risk is reduced, if ovulation is not triggered when the estradiol level or number of maturing follicles is excessive.
2. *Hyperstimulation syndrome:* It is an iatrogenic enlargement of the ovaries after ovulation induction with gonadotropin. In this due to increased vascular permeability occurring in luteal phase, fluid shift occurs from intravascular space to third space. It is seen more in young age, low body weight, PCOS and with high doses of gonadotropin.[1]
3. *Breast and ovarian cancer:* There have been no consistent reports of the relation between gonadotropin and carcinoma breast and ovary.
4. *Miscarriage:* In about 25% of patients on gonadotropin therapy, miscarriage can happen.

The gonadotropin therapy can be used independently. It can also be used with first-line drugs like clomiphene and letrozole, where less dose of gonadotropin is required. And it can also be combined with GnRH analogue to reduce the incidence of hyper-stimulation and OHSS by preventing premature LH surge.

INDUCTION OF OVULATION IN PCOS PATIENTS

In PCOS patients, first choice for ovulation induction in anovulatory patient is nonsteroidal selective estrogen receptor modulator, i.e. clomiphene citrate. Alternatively, other drugs like tamoxifen (SERM) or aromatase inhibitors (AI), i.e. letrozole, can be used. However, if resistance or failure of these drugs occurs, then one has no choice other than using gonadotropin injection. They are also needed in anovulatory patients when patient is not tolerating these drugs or there are serious side effects of these drugs.

The problem of PCOS patients with gonadotropins is their tendency for OHSS. This is due to the fact that they contain twice the number of FSH sensitive antral follicles. Due to this chronic low dose regime is employed where FSH started on day 3 at low dosage of 37.5–75 IU for 14 days in first cycle and 7 days in subsequent cycle. Thereafter, increments of 25–37.5 IU are given at weekly intervals until follicular development is initiated and it reaches the satisfactory size (20–22 mm) and then hCG can be given. Compared to the conventional step-up protocol, pregnancy rates are found to improve (40% vs 24%). Uniovulation was induced in more patients (74% vs 27%) and there was no OHSS and/or multiple pregnancies, which was prevalent (11% OHSS and 33% multiple pregnancies).[13]

To avoid multiple pregnancies, strict criteria are followed for administration of hCG as follows:

• The number of follicles greater than 14 mm should not be more than 3 and estradiol should be less than 1500 pg/mL.

In poorly responding PCOS patients, conventional step-up protocol may be tried where the gonadotropin is started at 150 IU and increased by 75 IU according to response.

Recently, some studies show better results regarding unifollicular ovulation with step-down regimes compared with low dose step-up protocols. It is suggested that pure FSH gives better results in cases where LH levels are high.

In short, following points should be taken into consideration when gonadotropins are to be used in PCOS patients:

1. Proper selection of the patient.
2. After failure or resistance to the first-line/alternative drugs.
3. Induction with gonadotropin care must be taken to avoid multifollicular development and adverse consequences like OHSS and multiple pregnancies.
4. Chronic low dose step-up protocol is safe in terms of monofollicular development and avoids complications like OHSS and multiple pregnancies.
5. GnRH antagonist protocol with GnRHa triggers for the follicular maturation nearly eliminates the risk of OHSS.
6. PCOS patients are usually started on a low dose to avoid hyperstimulation and if LH is raised then only FSH-containing preparations are used.
7. Lastly, women with PCOS should be followed closely during pregnancy as they may be at increased risk for the development of gestational diabetes mellitus, hypertension and other associated complications.

REFERENCES

1. Dr. Surveen Ghumman. Step by step ovulation induction book; Jaypee brothers (Delhi) and Anshan publications (UK) 2006; 6:84.
2. Broekmans FJ, Knauff EA, Valkenburg O, et al. PCOS according to the Rotterdam consensus criteria: change in prevalence among WHO - II anovulation and association with metabolic factors. BJOG .2006;113 (110):1210–7.
3. Stein IF, Leventhal ML. Amenorrhea associated with bilateral polycystic ovaries. Am J Obstet Gynecol. 1935;29:181–91.
4. Dr. Kamini A Rao. The infertility manual edited by Kamini and Divyashree , published by - The

health sciences publishers - Delhi | London and Jaypee publishers, Delhi. 4th edition 2018; Chapter 11 by Deepika Krishna: Page - 80 - 87. And Chapter 28 by Mekhla Dwarkanath : Page 249–255

5. The Rotterdam ESHRE/ASRM sponsored PCOS consensus workshop group: Fauser B, Tarlatzis B , Chang J, Azziz R et al. Revised 2003 consensus on diagnostic criteria and long term health risks related to polycystic ovarian syndrome (PCOS). Hum Reprod 2004;19:41–7.

6. Balen AH, Laven JSE, Tan SL, Dewailly D.Ultrasound assessment of polycystic ovary: international consensus definitions. Human Reprod Update 2003;9:505–14.

7. Dr. Surveen Ghumman - Step by step ovulation induction book ; Published by Jaypee brothers (Delhi) and Anshan publications (UK) in 2006;1:02.

8. Birch Peterson K, Pederson NG, Pederse AT, Lauritsen MP, Cour Freiesleben NL. Mono-ovulation in women with polycystic ovary syndrome: a clinical review on ovulation induction. Reprod Biomed Online. 2016;32: 563–83.

9. De Paula Guedes Neto E, Savaris RF, von Eye Corleta H, de Moraes GS, do Amaral Cristovam R, Lessey BA. Prospective, randomized comparison between raloxifene and clomiphene citrate for ovulation induction in polycystic ovary syndrome. Fertil steril. 2011;96(3):769–73.

10. ESHRE Capri Workshop Group. Mono-ovulatory cycles: a key goal in profertility programmes. Human Reprod Update. 2003;9(3):263–74.

11. Lan VTN, Norman RJ, Nhu GH, Tuan PH, Tuong HM. Ovulation induction using low-dose step-up rFSH in Vietnamese women with polycystic ovary syndrome. Reprod Biomed Online. 2009;18(4):516–21.

12. Hugues JN, Cedrin-Dumerin I, Avril C, Bulwa S, Herve-Fand-Uzan M. Sequential step up and step down regimen: An alternative method for ovulation induction with FSH in polycystic ovarian syndrome. Hum Reprod 1996;11:2581–4.

13. Homberg R, Levy T, Ben Rafael Z. A comparative prospective study of conventional regimen with chronic low dose administration of follicle stimulating hormone for anovulation associated with polycystic ovary syndrome. Fertil Steril 1995;63:729–33.

Ovulation Induction in PCOS: Letrozole

Himadri Bal, Umesh Sable

The genesis of the symptomatology of polycystic ovarian syndrome (PCOS) to a large extent stems from chronic anovulation. As a corollary, ovulation induction remains the basic management of PCOS. The drugs commonly used are clomiphene citrate, metformin and gonadotropins with clomiphene citrate being the first line of treatment. However, things are not always very smooth sailing with clomiphene. The problems with clomiphene citrate, basically arises from its anti-estrogenic effect interfering with the cervical mucus and proper development of the endometrium. Other side effects, though less than gonadotropins, are ovarian hyper-stimulation syndrome (OHSS) and multiple pregnancy. Hunt for safer alternatives led to the appearance of letrozole in the arena of ovulation induction in PCOS patients. In spite of the positive side of letrozole, it met with hurdles in its use for ovulation induction.

The history of letrozole as an ovulation induction drug is mired in some controversy. It was at the commencement of the new millennium (2000–2001) that aromatase inhibitors were brought into the realm of ovulation induction by two gentlemen, Robert Casper and Mohamed FM Mitwally working in Toronto General Hospital.[1] Letrozole was introduced as an alternative to clomiphene. Casper and Mitwally came to know of the aromatase inhibitor letrozole, which was being marketed by Novartis by the trade name Femara. This drug along with anastrozole, another aromatase inhibitor, were being used as adjuvant therapy in estrogen receptor positive metastatic breast cancer cases. Keeping in mind the mechanism of action of aromatase inhibitors, a pilot study was undertaken to test the efficacy of letrozole in ovulation induction and the scope of its use in clomiphene failure cases. The study was published in 2000.[2] The advantage of letrozole over clomiphene is that it causes single ovulation, there is no anti-estrogenic effect and not known to cause OHSS.

However, use of letrozole in ovulation induction was questioned in the annual meeting of the American Society of Reproductive Medicine in 2005. In this conference, a doctor from Montreal, Marinko Biljan, a reproductive endocrinologist, presented a paper in which he reported congenital anomalies in 150 babies delivered by infertile women treated with letrozole.[3] After this, all hell broke loose. Larger multi-centric studies were carried out to gauge the efficacy and safety of letrozole. Though subsequent studies could not substantiate the allegation of letrozole being teratogenic, its use for ovulation induction was shunned the world over. Research data showed that off-springs of letrozole induction were not at higher risk of developing cardiac, locomotive or overall congenital malformations.[4] In spite of these findings, letrozole was being used as an off-label drug or only for research purposes. It was not approved for ovulation induction. The manufacture and sale of letrozole was banned in India in 2011(Gazette notification dated 12th October 2011).

Five years later after various studies to assess the risk profile of letrozole, the Indian Council of Medical Research (ICMR) recommended that letrozole was safe and can be used for infertility treatment. Based on the ICMR recommendation, the Government of India withdrew the ban on letrozole in 2017 (Gazette notification dated 17th February 2017).

Pharmacology of Letrozole

Letrozole is an antifungal triazole derivative which acts as aromatase inhibitor. Aromatase is a microsomal cytochrome P450 hemoprotein containing enzyme (P450 arom), the product of the CYP19 gene. It catalyzes the conversion of C-19 steroids, that is androgens (androstenedione, testosterone, dehydroepiandrosterone) to C-18 steroids, which are estrogens (estrone, estradiol, estriol, respectively). Inhibition of the aromatase enzyme leads to hypoestrogenemia, which in turn stimulates the hypothalamic–pituitary–ovarian axis leading to the release of FSH from the pituitary. The released FSH leads to the stimulation of follicular growth and ovulation. Letrozole is completely absorbed on oral administration, metabolized in the liver and excreted by the kidneys. Its half-life is about 45 hours. The advantages of letrozole are:

- It does not have any estrogen receptor depleting action and thus its action is more physiological.
- A short half-life of 45 hours vis-à-vis 5 days to 3 weeks of clomiphene
- This relative early clearance makes the drug safer with less chance of side effects.
- It is known to cause monofollicular development.

Dosage and Method of Administration

1. Letrozole is administered orally. The starting dose is 2.5 mg once daily for 5 days, usually starting from day 3 of the cycle. The dose can be gradually increased to 5 mg/day, and then to a maximum dose of 7.5 mg/day depending on the response. Generally, a 5 mg dose is sufficient for ovulation induction.
2. Letrozole can also be combined with gonadotropins.

Results

The efficacy of letrozole has varied in different studies. There are articles where some have shown no difference from clomiphene;[5] others quoted 86% ovulation rate and 20% pregnancy rate.[6]

Comparison to Clomiphene

According to the WHO classification of anovulation, Type II or normogonadotropic anovulation is one of the prominent causes of infertility. PCOS constitutes 90% of these Type II cases.[7] Hence ovulation induction remains the cornerstone of treatment of infertility in PCOS patients.

Till date, clomiphene remains the most widely used first-line drug for ovulation induction. It is a nonsteroidal selective estrogen receptor modulator having both estrogenic and anti-estrogenic effects. Clomiphene leads to increased secretion of gonadotropin from the pituitary by binding to the estrogen receptors (ERs) in the hypothalamus. This blocks the negative feedback effect of peripheral estradiol on the hypothalamus, thus leading to increased secretion of FSH from the pituitary gland and thereby stimulating folliculogenesis. Aromatase inhibitors like letrozole, on the contrary, have no ER blocking effect. They induce a peripheral hypoestrogenic state by inhibiting the conversion of androgens to estrogens in the steroidogenic pathway. This peripheral estrogen deficiency directly stimulates the hypothalamic release of GnRH leading to FSH secretion from the pituitary which in turn stimulates follicle growth. Therefore, the mechanism of action of letrozole is more physiological. It maintains the primacy of the dominant follicle. Since there is no ER blocking effect, the dominant follicle as it grows, peripheral estrogen levels keep rising and normal physiologic suppression of FSH and atresia of smaller follicles is maintained. This prevents multiple ovulation and, therefore, multiple pregnancies and also reduces the chances of OHSS.

The anti-estrogenic action of clomiphene affects the endometrium leading to the dissociation of the simultaneous harmonious progression of the endometrial and ovarian cycle. This disconnect, affects the implantation of the fertilized ovum leading to the discrepancy between the ovulation rates and pregnancy rates after clomiphene treatment. Aromatase inhibitors do not show this anomaly. Moreover, aromatase inhibitors, having short half-lives, do not stay-on in the system to exert any adverse effect on estrogen target tissues, namely endometrium and cervical mucus.

Studies on letrozole use in clomiphene resistant cases have shown ovulation rates of 50–90% and pregnancy rates of 10–40%.[8] In 2014, a large multicentric double blind randomized control study comparing the cumulative live birth rates of letrozole and clomiphene in cases of PCOS with anovulatory infertility was published in the New England Journal of Medicine. It clearly showed letrozole had an edge over clomiphene in the live birth rates (27.5% and 19.1% in favor of letrozole).[9]

As regards fetal safety is concerned, FDA categorises letrozole as pregnancy category 'D' and clomiphene as category 'X' drug. So both the drugs when exposed during organo-genesis in animal models are found to be teratogenic.[10] It is a different matter that clinically, when used for ovulation induction and if it is successful, both the drugs are excreted out of the system long before commencement of organogenesis.

To conclude, different studies have come up with different recommendations on letrozole use for ovulation induction. Some

recommend it as a first-line treatment option, others advocate it as a second-line drug in clomiphene resistant cases.

The advantages of letrozole over clomiphene put forward are:

- Less chance of multiple pregnancy and abortions.
- Does not interfere with the endometrial thickness or the cervical mucus.
- Side effects, like OHSS, or menopausal symptoms like hot flushes which are sometimes seen with clomiphene, are almost non-existent with letrozole.
- Should be considered as first-line drug in obese women.

However, whether at this point, letrozole can be labeled as the first-line treatment for anovulatory infertility in PCOS is debatable. The points in favor of this view point are studies supporting letrozole have been carried out in selected groups in selective geo-graphical areas and, therefore, global validation lacking. Letrozole resistance or failure has still not been conclusively defined.[11] Hence it is recommended that further studies are required to validate the efficacy and superiority of letrozole.

REFERENCES

1. Mitwally MF, Casper RF. Aromatase Inhibition: A novel method of ovulation induction in women with polycystic ovarian syndrome. Reprod Technol. 2000; 10:244–247.
2. Mitwally MF, Casper RF. Use of an aromatase inhibitor for induction of ovulation in patients with an inadequate response to clomiphene citrate. Fertil Steril. 2000;75:305–309.
3. Biljan MM, Hemmings R, Brassard N. The outcome of 150 babies following the treatment with letrozole or letrozole and gonadotropins. Fertil Steril. 2005;84(Suppl 1):S95.
4. Casper RF, Mitwally MF. A historical perspective of aromatase inhibitors for ovulation induction. Fertil Steril. 2012;98:1352–1355.
5. Mary Angel, Seetesh Ghose, Mamata Gowda. A randomized trial comparing the ovulation induction efficacy of clomiphene citrate and letrozole. J Nat Sci Biol Med 2014;5(2):450–452.

6. Zeinalzadeh M, Basirat Z, Esmailpour M. Efficacy of letrozole in ovulation induction compared to that of clomiphene citrate in patient with polycystic ovarian syndrome. The Journal of reproductive medicine 2010;55(1-2):36–40.

7. ESHRE Capri Workshop Group. Health and fertility in World Health Organization group 2 anovulatory women. Hum Reprod Update 2012; 18:586–599.

8. Requena A, Herrero J, Landeras J, et al. Use of letrozole in assisted reproduction: a systematic review and meta-analysis. Hum Reprod Update 2008; 14:571–582.

9. Richard S. Legro, Robert G. Brzyski, Michael P. Diamond,et al. Letrozole versus Clomiphene for Infertility in the Polycystic Ovary Syndrome. N Engl J Med 2014; 371:119–129.

10. Reefhuis J, Honein MA, Schieve LA, Rasmussen SA. Use of clomiphene citrate and birth defects, National Birth Defects Prevention Study, 1997-2005. Hum Reprod 2011;26:451–457.

11. Stefano Palomba. Aromatase Inhibitors for Ovulation Induction. The Journal of Clinical Endocrinology & Metabolism. 2015; 100(5):1742–1747.

18

Preventing and Managing Ovarian Hyperstimulation Syndrome

Hemant Deshpande, Suyajan D Joshi, Priyanka Dahiya

INTRODUCTION

Ovarian hyperstimulation syndrome (OHSS) is an iatrogenic complication occurring as a result of controlled ovarian stimulation for infertility treatment. It is almost always a result of human chorionic gonadotropin (hCG) administration in a susceptible patient or during early pregnancy which leads to local and systemic increase in capillary permeability resulting in intravascular volume depletion and third space fluid accumulation (presenting as ascites, pleural effusion) along with direct stimulatory effect of gonadotropins resulting in ovarian enlargement.

PATHOPHYSIOLOGY

Multiple studies have demonstrated complex interplay between immune and reproductive systems as a consequence of sharing certain lymphohematopoietic cytokines and their receptors in prediction and pathogenesis of OHSS.[1] With the exposure of hyperstimulated ovaries to hCG there is production of proinflammatory mediators which are involved in the pathogenesis and their local and systemic effects including increased vascular permeability and a prothrombotic effect are responsible for the clinical features of OHSS. Various factors postulated are: Vascular permeability factor, cytokines, vascular endothelial growth factor (VEGF), interleukins, and immunoreactive endothelins.

Large amounts of vascular permeability factor (VPF) demonstrated in follicular fluid compared with serum or peritoneal fluid of patients undergoing controlled ovarian hyperstimulation is suggestive of VPF being responsible for acute, third space fluid sequestration.[2] Significant increase in permeability of endothelial cells *in vitro* has been demonstrated in follicular fluid and peritoneal fluid obtained from these patients.[3] The expression of VPF-mRNA in human luteinized granulosa cells is dose and time dependant which is enhanced by hCG.[4] It has been further proposed that the elevated levels of IL-2, IL-6, IL-8 and TNF as well as low levels of nitrites demonstrated in the ascitic fluid from OHSS patients could be involved in mediating the increased permeability in OHSS through nitric oxide system.[5] Abramov, et al. studied that high plasma inflammatory cytokines concentrations (IL-1, IL-6, TNF) which were recorded at time of admissions in cases of severe OHSS dropped to normal values with significant clinical improvement.[6] They could also demonstrate statistically significant correlation between plasma cytokine concentration and leukocytosis, raised hematocrit and increased estradiol levels. Angiogenin plays a vital role in formation of neovascularization further responsible for development of OHSS.[7] VEGF also has a vital role to play in cyclic ovarian angiogenesis and has a strong ability to increase membrane permeabilty. VEGF-A concentrations have been demonstrated to be elevated following hCG administration and in women with or at risk of OHSS.[39,40]

Erythrocyte aggregation causes capillary leak and it has been enhanced in peripheral venous blood of patients with COH and OHSS.[8] Resetting of plasma osmotic threshold for arginine vasopressin secretion to a lower level during superovulation was observed by Evbuomwan, et al.[9] Women with severe OHSS develop hypovolemia, with a loss of 20% of their calculated blood volume in the acute phase of OHSS. Along with this hypovolemia, there is reduced serum osmolality and sodium. This paradoxical combination of hypovolemia and hypo-osmolality is a result of 'reset' of the osmotic thresholds of vasopressin and thirst to lower osmolality and sodium levels as these subjects remain able to concentrate/dilute their urine around the new, lower, level of osmolality. The parallel resetting of the osmotic thresholds is thought to explain the observed decrease in serum osmolality and sodium as opposed to electrolyte losses.

It is marked by massive bilateral cystic ovarian enlargement, increased stromal edema, interspersed with multiple hemorrhagic follicular and theca-lutein cysts, areas of cortical necrosis and neovascularization. Second pathological phenomenon as a result of increased capillary permeability is that of acute body fluid shifts, resulting in ascites and pleural effusion. Figure 18.1 summarizes the pathophysiology of OHSS.

PRESENTATIONS OF OHSS

a. *Depending upon etiology—iatrogenic and spontaneous*: In iatrogenic form of OHSS, the follicular recruitment and enlargement occur during ovarian stimulation with exogenous FSH while in spontaneous form, the follicular recruitment occurs later through stimulation of FSH receptor through pregnancy-derived hCG. Then massive luteinization of enlarged stimulated ovaries starts, inducing the release of vasoactive mediators leading to clinical symptoms.

b. *Depending upon the time of presentation following trigger injection—early and late OHSS*: 'Early' OHSS usually presents within 7–9 days of the hCG injection and reflects excessive ovarian response and precipitating effect of exogenous hCG administered for final follicular maturation. 'Late' OHSS typically presents 10 or more days after the hCG injection and reflects the endogenous hCG derived from an early pregnancy. Late OHSS is more severe and prolonged than the early form of OHSS.

INCIDENCE

The incidence varies widely among different centers due to different definitions for grades of severity. The incidence reported for mild OHSS is 20–33%[11] of IVF cycles, combined for

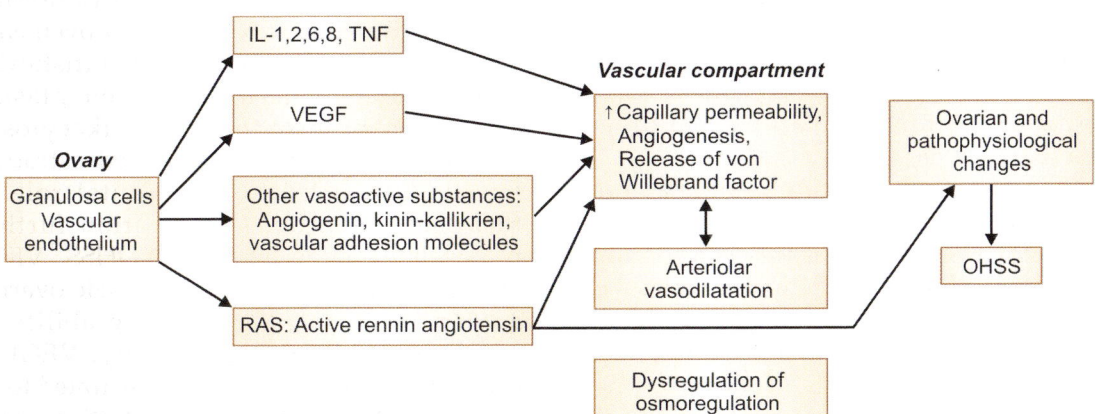

Fig. 18.1: Pathophysiology of OHSS[10]

moderate to severe to be 3.1–8%[12] of IVF cycles but can be as high as 20% in high-risk women.[12,38] Treatments involving greater degrees of ovarian stimulation are associated with a higher incidence.

Factors influencing the incidence are:

a. *Age:* Younger women are at high risk as compared to older women.

b. *Body mass index:* Contradictory reports have been published regarding correlation between lean body mass and OHSS. Low body weight is considered to be a risk factor.

c. *Etiology of infertility:* It has been observed equally in both primary and secondary infertility cases,[13] and although the duration of infertility has no influence on occurrence of OHSS.[14] Women who have previously developed OHSS are at increased risk of subsequent development.[15]

d. *Ovarian stimulation protocols:* Higher incidence of OHSS is observed after combined use of GnRH-agonist/HMG for COH.[16] Although no relationship has been demonstrated between the dose of gonadotropin administered and incidence of OHSS. The risk with use of FSH and HMG is similar. The use of recombinant FSH does not eliminate the risk of developing OHSS. However, the risk of severe form is rare with clomiphene citrate or monofollicular ovulation induction with gonadotropins. Higher incidence is reported after use of hCG for luteal support. In cases who are at high risk, intramuscular/vaginal progesterone may be given instead.

Evidence from meta-analysis[17] also shows a reduced risk of OHSS in IVF cycles employing gonadotropin-releasing hormone (GnRH) antagonists compared with cycles where GnRH agonists are used as part of the regimen for controlled ovarian hyperstimulation.

e. *Conception cycles:* Frequency of OHSS is higher (four times) in pregnancy than in non-pregnancy cycles.[18] The duration of OHSS is longer and its manifestation more severe when the pregnancy ensures. It is still grave in cycles that result in multiple pregnancy, highlighting the role of endogenous hCG.

f. Women with PCOS, increased antral follicle count (AFC) or high levels of anti-Müllerian hormone (AMH) are at an increased risk of OHSS.

CLASSIFICATION OF OHSS

Several classifications have been proposed for classifying the severity of OHSS,[19-22] with no clear agreement between investigators. Table 18.1 summarizes the RCOG classification of severity of PCOS.

DIAGNOSIS

There are no specific symptoms of OHSS and no diagnostic tests for the condition. A typical patient presents with abdominal distension and discomfort with history of trigger injection used to promote final follicular maturation prior to oocyte retrieval. There may be history of an excessive ovarian response to stimulation in past, but the absence of such a history does not necessarily rule out OHSS. Careful assessment by an experienced clinician, good history along with certain investigations is desirous for diagnosis and assessing the severity of condition. Relevant history from a woman suspected to be suffering from OHSS must include; time of onset of symptoms relative to trigger, medication used for trigger, number of follicles on final monitoring scan, number of eggs collected and history of polycystic ovary syndrome.

CLINICAL FEATURES

1. Abdominal bloating/distension
2. Abdominal discomfort/pain
3. Nausea and vomiting
4. Breathlessness

TABLE 18.1: Proposed RCOG classification of severity of OHSS

Severity	Clinical features
Mild OHSS	Abdominal bloating
	Mild abdominal pain
	Ovarian size usually <8 cm^3
Moderate OHSS	Moderate abdominal pain
	Nausea ± vomiting
	Ultrasound evidence of ascites
	Ovarian size usually 8–12 cm^3
Severe OHSS	Clinical ascites (±hydrothorax)
	Oliguria (<300 mL/day or <30 mL/hour)
	Hematocrit >0.45
	Hyponatremia (sodium <135 mmol/L)
	Hypo-osmolality (osmolality <282 mOsm/kg)
	Hyperkalemia (potassium >5 mmol/L)
	Hypoproteinemia (serum albumin <35 g/L)
	Ovarian size usually >12 cm^3
Critical OHSS	Tense ascites/large hydrothorax
	Hematocrit >0.55
	White cell count >25000/mL
	Oliguria/anuria
	Thromboembolism
	Acute respiratory distress syndrome

#In cases of ART, the ovarian size may not correlate with severity of OHSS due to the effect of follicular aspiration. Women having any features of severe or critical OHSS, should be classified in that category.

5. Reduced urine output
6. Leg swelling, vulval swelling
7. Associated comorbidities such as thrombosis

Clinical examination should include body weight, abdominal examination (including girth, degree of distension, palpable ovaries, presence or absence of ascites, tenderness), heart rate, blood pressure, chest examination, and assessment of hydration. Important differential diagnoses include ectopic pregnancy, intra-abdominal hemorrhage, appendicitis, complicated ovarian cyst (torsion, hemorrhage), pelvic infection/abscess and bowel perforation.

LABORATORY INVESTIGATIONS

1. Full blood count: Hemoglobin, hematocrit, WBC to assess hemoconcentration
2. CRP (severity)
3. Blood urea, serum electrolytes (hyponatremia and hyperkalemia)
4. Serum osmolality (hypo-osmolality)
5. Liver function tests (elevated enzymes, reduced albumin)
6. Serum β-hCG (to determine outcome of treatment cycle, if appropriate)
7. Baseline clotting studies (elevated fibrinogen, reduced antithrombin)
8. Pelvic ultrasound (ovarian size, pelvic/abdominal free fluid, color Doppler to rule out suspected ovarian torsion
9. Chest X-ray and ultrasonography, if respiratory symptoms are present.
10. *Others:* ECG, D-dimer, computerized tomography pulmonary angiogram (CTPA) or ventilation/perfusion (V/Q) scan, arterial blood gas analysis.

Elevated hematocrit, reduced serum osmolality along with hyponatremia is indicative of OHSS.[23]

TREATMENT

Initial assessment is crucial to establish the diagnosis and assess the severity of OHSS.

Outpatient management is appropriate for women with mild or moderate OHSS after a written informed consent about their condition. Paracetamol and oral opiates may be given for pain relief. Nonsteroidal anti-inflammatory drugs (NSAIDs) should be avoided as they may compromise renal function in women with OHSS.[24] Patients should be encouraged to drink to thirst rather than excess.[25] Fluid intake of at least 1 litre/day should be advised as it is the most physiological approach to replace volume avoiding the risk of hypervolemia and worsening ascites that may occur with vigorous intravenous therapy. Progesterone luteal support is continued and patient is reviewed every 2–3 days. Urgent review is needed, if there is worsening of pain, increasing abdominal distension, shortness of breath or a subjective impression of reduced urine output (less than 1000 mL/24 hours). In case the severity of OHSS is worsening, the baseline laboratory investigations should be repeated. Hematocrit is a very useful tool to assess the degree of intravascular volume depletion. In most women, the condition resolves over a period of 7–10 days.[26] In absence of pregnancy, recovery is usually complete by the time of the withdrawal bleed, but if conception occurs, worsening of OHSS may occur under effect of endogenous hCG.

Inpatient care is needed for worsening moderate OHSS and severe cases. Hospital admission should be considered for women who are unable to achieve satisfactory pain control or maintain adequate fluid intake due to nausea and show signs of worsening OHSS despite outpatient intervention. Antiemetics along with analgesics (paracetamol, opiates) are given. Nausea is related to accumulation of ascites, so measures to abdominal distension should help. Patients should be encouraged for hydration therapy via oral route. Where oral intake cannot be maintained, IV crystalloids such as normal saline 2–3 L/day, guided by a strict fluid balance chart should be given. Women with persistent hemoconcentration and/or urine output <0.5 mL/kg/hr may benefit from colloids like human albumin, 6% hydroxyethyl starch (HES), dextran, mannitol and Haemacel. Diuretics must be avoided as they deplete the intravascular volume. They may have a role with careful hemodynamic monitoring in cases where oliguria persist despite adequate intravascular volume expansion and a normal intra-abdominal pressure. Daily assessment is mandatory in admitted cases. LMWH prophylaxis should be given in those admitted with severe or critical OHSS. Thrombo-prophylaxis may be in form of full-length venous support stockings and prophylactic heparin or intermittent pneumatic compression device. The duration of LMWH prophylaxis should be according to patient risk factors and outcome of treatment. The risk of thrombosis persists in first trimester, in women who conceive. The clinician must balance the risks and benefits of heparin prophylaxis until the end of first trimester,[30,31] or even longer, depending upon the course of OHSS. Thrombo-prophylaxis may be discontinued in women who do not conceive with resolution of the condition. Paracentesis is indicated, if there is significant discomfort or respiratory compromise due to severe abdominal distension. Relief from intra-abdominal pressure may promote renal perfusion and improve urine output in cases with persistent oliguria despite adequate volume replacement. It is performed in a controlled manner (to avoid cardiovascular collapse resulting from massive fluid shifts) under ultrasound guidance (to avoid inadvertent puncture of vascular ovaries distended by large luteal cysts) abdominally or vaginally with continuous pulse and blood pressure monitoring with IV colloids administration. Paracentesis may suffice to resolve hydro-thorax; however, if it persist, may be drained directly. Surgical intervention may be needed at the hands of experienced surgeon following careful assessment in cases of adnexal torsion or conincidental problems like ovarian rupture or ectopic pregnancy, requiring surgery. Untwisting of the twisted adnexa followed by observation of improved color at laparoscopy or laparotomy is associated with a favorable prognosis of ovarian function. In rare cases of critical OHSS, termination of pregnancy in the situation of progressive thrombosis despite anticoagulation,[32] bilateral oophorectomy for intractable OHSS[33] have been reported.

Inpatient monitoring of women with OHSS is mandatory to note any progression or regression in severity of the disease process and to identify any complications at the earliest. Daily record of body weight, abdominal girth, and fluid intake and output should be maintained, along with full blood count, serum electrolytes, hematocrit, osmolality and liver function tests. Depending on the clinical features, other investigations like arterial blood gases, ECG, chest skiagram may be required. Worsening of OHSS may be picked up with signs of weight gain, increasing abdominal girth, oliguria with positive fluid balance and elevated hematocrit. Conversely, recovery is signalled by a diuresis, normalization of hematocrit and a reduction in abdominal girth and body weight.[27,28] C-reactive protein levels have been shown to correlate with other markers of OHSS such as abdominal girth and weight, and may have a role in monitoring severity.[29]

Intensive care is needed in critical cases of OHSS or if specific complications like ARDS, renal failure, thromboembolism ensue. More frequent assessment is needed in critical OHSS cases and those with complications. Severe cases of OHSS where initial crystalloid and colloid therapy fails to correct dehydration and hemoconcentration also requires more frequent assessment and thus ICU care.

COMPLICATIONS OF OHSS

a. *Vascular complications:* Incidence of thrombosis is 0.7–10%, with an apparent preponderance of upper body sites and frequent involvement of arterial system.[30,31] Hemoconcentration and severe leukocytosis are considered risk factors for thromboembolic diseases in patients with OHSS. Thus heparin should be considered in all patients to prevent thromboembolism. Unusual neurological symptoms should raise the possibility of a thrombotic episode. Serious cerebrovascular thrombosis resulting in hemiparesis, central retinal artery occlusion, cerebral infarction and myocardial infarction have been reported in literature.

b. Febrile morbidity

c. Liver dysfunction

d. *Respiratory complications* may present with variety of signs and symptoms in OHSS. Dyspnea and tachypneas are most common symptoms. Local pneumonia, adult respiratory distress syndrome, pulmonary embolism, and pleural effusion may develop in severe or critical cases of OHSS.

e. Benign intracranial tension

f. *Renal complications:* Prerenal failure due to hypovolemia secondary to fluid transudation in peritoneal cavity may occur.

g. *Gastrointestinal complications:* Mesenteric resection after mesenteric artery occlusion, duodenal ulcer perforation, have been reported.

   Obstetrical complications: A higher incidence of pre-eclampsia (21.2%) and prematurity (36%) has been demonstrated in OHSS pregnancies compared with a control group of IVF pregnancies without OHSS.[34,35] The incidences of multiple pregnancies were almost similar between the two groups. The risk of miscarriage in pregnancies arising from assisted reproduction cycles complicated by OHSS does not rise compared to cycles without OHSS.[36,37] Some reports have suggested an increased rate of preclinical pregnancy loss in women with early, but not late, OHSS.[37]

h. Prolonged hospitalization

PREVENTION OF OHSS

Although there is no perfect strategy which can completely eliminate OHSS. Factors which we can take into consideration in order to reduce its incidence are:

1. Identifying the 'At Risk' Women

For a safe or controlled ovarian stimulation, it is important to define the at risk population. Table 18.2 enlists various risk factors for developing OHSS. Hormonal markers are being employed in predicting the ovarian response to stimulation. AMH with its low inter- and intracycle variability can identify normal responders to controlled ovarian stimulation and at risk women with a success rate of 98%.[41] Antral follicle count (AFC) and basal serum AMH, equally predict the excessive response to COS.[42,43] A combination of ≥18 follicles on ultrasound (diameter ≥11 mm) and E2 ≥5000 ng/L on the day of hCG trigger has been found to be more useful (sensitivity 83%, specificity 84%) than E2 concentrations alone in the prediction of severe OHSS.[44]

2. Primary Prevention

It can be done by modifying the treatment regimens to curtail over excessive ovarian response.

Aiming at unifollicular ovulation especially in women with PCOS through ovulation induction definitely will reduce the risk of OHSS.

TABLE 18.2: Risk factors for developing OHSS

Young (age <30 years)
Polycystic ovaries
High serum estradiol (ART >4000 pg/ml, OI >1700 pg/ml)
Multiple stimulated follicles (ART >20, AI >6)
Necklace sign
Pregnancy
hCG luteal support
GnRH down regulatory protocol
High serum AMH levels

Reducing gonadotropin dose: Evidence suggests that the minimum gonadotropin dose should be used for OI. So a 'step-up' regimen is favourable over a 'step-down' regimen. In the 'step-up' regimen, ovarian stimulation is initiated with a low dose of FSH (i.e. 75 IU), which is subsequently increased every 7 days until an ovarian response is noted. This dose is then continued until the criteria for an ovulatory trigger are met.[45,46] This is advantageous over other low dose/step-down protocols as it is associated with a lower risk of OHSS, cycle cancellation, and a higher rate of unifollicular development. In a 'step-down' regimen, a higher starting FSH dose is used which is downtitrated based on ovarian response.[47,48] Many studies have shown that the method of stimulation (chronic low dose, step-up or step-down) is more important as a risk factor as compared with the type of injectable gonadotropin used.

Avoiding adjunct GnRH-a: Use of gonadotropin-releasing hormone agonist (GnRH-a) either as a long or short protocol in conjunction with controlled ovarian hyperstimulation affects the risk of OHSS. Both these protocols abolish the mid-cycle LH surge which drives more follicles to maturation with consequent rise in estradiol value, hence more risk of OHSS. In contrast, cycles without GnRH-a suppression a significant LH surge limits the continued gonadotropin stimulation and hence lesser risk of OHSS.

Reducing the gonadotropin duration by incorporating 'mild' stimulation protocols which delay the administration of FSH till the mid or late follicular phase. The addition of GnRH antagonists for late cycle suppression of gonadotropin release is beneficial as it results in improved clinical outcomes, a lower risk of OHSS and multiple pregnancies.

Adjuvant metformin therapy: Metformin inhibits the secretion of vasoactive molecules, such as VEGF, during OI and thereby modulates vascular permeability.[49] Metformin reduces the risk of OHSS by 63% and increases the clinical pregnancy rate without an effect on live birth rates.[50] A daily dose between 1000 and 2000 mg at least 2 months prior to COS is recommended for the purpose of preventing OHSS.[51-53]

Individualizing IVF treatment regimens: An algorithm was formulated based on age, AFC, and FSH to calculate the FSH starting dose. This accurately predicts the ovarian sensitivity and accounts for 30% of the variability of ovaries to FSH. The starting FSH dose or tailored GnRH antagonist protocol can then be decided based on an algorithm of these biomarkers.

Use of GnRH antagonists instead of agonists to prevent premature LH surge; reduction in dose of hCG; use of LH or GnRH-a in place of hCG for trigger are effective in preventing OHSS.

3. Secondary Prevention

It aims to prevent progression to OHSS.

Cycle cancellation: Cycle cancellation and withholding of hCG are the only definite methods of preventing OHSS.[56,57]

Coasting: An extension of step-down concept is 'coasting' which helps to prevent or reduce the risk of OHSS by altering the capacity of granulosa cells to produce VEGF, thus the cycle outcome is not compromised. It is a preventative strategy by which gonadotropins are withdrawn when a certain E2 concentration and/or a critical number of follicles are reached. The hCG trigger is delayed until E2 levels significantly decrease or plateau. Once the E2 reaches a 'safe' level, hCG is administered followed by oocyte retrieval and embryo transfer or freezing depending on the E2 concentration.[54] No significant effect on live birth rates and clinical pregnancy rates has been found by coasting.

Cryopreservation of embryos: In this procedure, COS and subsequent oocyte retrieval is performed followed by the cryopreserving the embryos. These cryopreserved embryos are then transferred during an unstimulated IVF cycle where the ovarian response to hCG has normalized. Recent evidence, however, strongly supports the use of a GnRHa trigger followed by cryopreservation as being the most effective method in preventing OHSS.[55] With the advent of vitrification, there is strong evidence to suggest that cryopreservation has better pregnancy rates (32% increase) than fresh embryo transfer.

Preventive infusion of colloids (HES) at time of oocyte retrieval has also been noted to reduce the incidence of OHSS.

4. Alternative Methods

Preventive infusion of colloids (HES) at time of oocyte retrieval has also been noted to reduce the incidence of OHSS by binding to and deactivating the vasoactive mediators of OHSS. Cabergoline is a dopamine antagonist which prevents the excessive increase in VEGF-mediated vascular permeability through its antiangiogenic properties. Treatment be commenced on the day of hCG trigger at a dose of 0.5 mg for 8 days.

REFERENCES

1. Ben-Rafael Z, Orvieto R. cytokine involvement in reproduction. Fertil Steril 1992;58:1093–9.

2. Krasnow JS, Berga SL, Guzick DS, et al. Vascular permeability factor and vascular endothelial growth factor in ovarian hyperstimulation syndrome: a preliminary report. Fertil Steril 1996; 65:552–5.

3. Goldman MP, Pedram A, Dominguez CE et al. Increased capillary permeability induced by human follicular fluid: a hypothesis for an ovarian origin of hyperstimulation syndrome. Fertil Steril 1995;63:268–72.

4. Neulen J, Yan Z, Raczek S, et al. Human chorionic gonadotrophin dependant expression of vascular endothelial growth factor/vascular permeability factor in human granulose cells : importance in ovarian hyperstimulation syndrome. J Clin Endocrinol Metab 1995;80:1967–71.

5. Revel A, Barak V, Lavy Y, et al. Characterization of intraperitoneal cytokines and nitrites in women with severe ovarian hyperstimulation syndrome. Fertil Steril 1996;66:66–71.

6. Abramov Y, Schenker JG, Lewin A, et al. Plasma inflammatory cytokines correlate to the ovarian hyperstimulation syndrome. HumReprod 1996; 11:1381–6.

7. Aboulghar MA,Mansour RT, Serour GI, et al. Elevated levels of Angiogenin in serum and ascetic fluid from patients with severe ovarian hyperstimulation syndrome. Hum Reprod 1998; 13:2068–71.

8. Levin I, Gamzu R, Hasson Y, et al. Increased erythrocyte aggregation in ovarian hyper-stimulation syndrome: a possible contributing factor in pathophysiology of this disease. Hum Reprod 2004; 19:1076–80.

9. Evbuomwan IO, Davison JM, Baylis PM, et al. Altered osmotic thresholds for arginine vasopressin secretion and thirst during superovulation and in ovarian hyperstimulation syndrome : relevance to the pathophysiology of OHSS. Fertil Steril 2001;75:933–41.

10. Delvigne A. The epidemiology and pathophysio-logy of ovarian hyperstimulation syndrome in assisted reproductive technologies : Quality and safety. New York: Parthenon publishing, 2004: 149–62.

11. Mathur RS, Akande AV, Keay SD, et al. Distinction between early and late ovarian hyperstimulation syndrome. Fertil Steril 2000;73: 901–7.

12. Delvigne A,Rozenberg S. Epidemiology and prevention of ovarian hyperstimulation syndrome (OHSS): a review. Hum Reprod Update 2002;8:559–77.

13. Delvigne A. Epidemiology and pathophysiology of ovarian hyperstimulation syndrome. In Gerris J, Olivennes F, de Sutter P, eds. Assited Reproductive Technologies: Quality and safety. New York: Parthenon publishing, 2004:149–62.

14. Navot D, Relou A, Birkenfeld A, et al. Risk factors and prognostic variables in ovarian hyperstimulation syndrome. Am J Obstet Gynaecol 1988;159:210–15.

15. Delvigne A, Dubois M, Battheu B, et al. The ovarian hyperstimulation syndrome in in-vitro fertilization: A Belgian muticenter study. II. Multiple discriminant analysis for risk prediction. Hum Reprod 1993;8:1361–6.

16. Golan A, Ron-El R, Herman A, et al. Ovarian hyperstimulation syndrome following D-Trp-6 luteinizing hormone releasing hormone micro-capsules and menotrophin for in-vitro fertilization. Fertil Steril 1988;50:912–16.

17. Al-Inany HG, Youssef MA, Aboulghar M, Broekmans F, Sterrenburg M, Smit J, et al. GnRH antagonists are safer than agonists: an update of a Cochrane review. Hum Reprod Update 2011;17:435.

18. Rizk B. Ovarian hyperstimulation syndrome. In Studd J, ed. Progress in Obstetrics and Gyaecology. Edinburgh: Churchill livingstone, 1993;11:311–49.

19. Schenker JG, Weinstein D. Ovarian hyper-stimulation syndrome: a current survey. Fertil Steril 1978;30:255–68.

20. Golan A, Ron-el R, Herman A, SofferY, Weinraub Z, Caspi E. Ovarian hyperstimulation syndrome: an update review. Obstet Gynecol Surv 1989;44:430–40.

21. Navot D, Bergh PA, Laufer N. Ovarian hyper-stimulation syndrome in novel reproductive technologies: prevention and treatment. Fertil Steril 1992;58:249–61.

22. Mathur R, Evbuomwan I, Jenkins J. Prevention and management of ovarian hyperstimulation syndrome. Curr Obstet Gynaecol 2005;15:132–8.

23. Evbuomwan I. The role of osmoregulation in the pathophysiology and management of severe ovarian hyperstimulation syndrome. Hum Fertil (Camb) 2013; 16:162–7.

24. Balasch J, Carmona F, Llach J,Arroyo V, Jové I,Vanrell JA. Acute prerenal failure and liver dysfunction in a patient with severe ovarian hyperstimulation syndrome. Hum Reprod 1990;5:348–51.

25. Evbuomwan I. The role of osmoregulation in the pathophysiology and management of severe ovarian hyperstimulation syndrome. Hum Fertil (Camb) 2013; 16:162–7.

26. Nouri K,Tempfer CB, Lenart C,Windischbauer L,Walch K, Promberger R,et al.Predictive factors for recovery time in patients suffering from severe OHSS. Reprod Biol Endocrinol 2014;12:59.

27. Practice Committee of the American Society for Reproductive Medicine. Ovarian hyperstimula-tion syndrome. Fertil Steril 2008;90 Suppl 5: S188–93.

28. Fábregues F, Balasch J, Manau D, Jiménez W, Arroyo V, Creus M, et al. Haematocrit, leukocyte and platelet counts and the severity of the

ovarian hyperstimulation syndrome. Hum Reprod 1998;13:2406–10.

29. Nowicka MA, Fritz-Rdzanek A, Grzybowski W, Walecka I, Niemiec KT,JakimiukAJ.C-reactive protein as the indicator of severity in ovarian hyperstimulation syndrome. Gynecol Endocrinol 2010;26:399–403.

30. Royal College of Obstetricians and Gynaecologists. Reducing the Risk of Venous Thromboembolism during Pregnancy and the Puerperium. Green-top Guideline No. 37a. London: RCOG; 2015.

31. ESHRE CapriWorkshop Group.Venous thromboembolism in women: a specific reproductive health risk. Hum Reprod Update 2013;19:471–82.

32. Cupisti S, Emran J, Mueller A, Dittrich R, Beckmann MW, Binder H. Course of ovarian hyperstimulation syndrome in 19 intact twin pregnancies after assisted reproduction techniques, with a case report of severe thromboembolism. Twin Res Hum Genet 2006;9:691–6.

33. Amarin ZO. Bilateral partial oophorectomy in the management of severe ovarian hyperstimulation syndrome. An aggressive, but perhaps life-saving procedure. Hum Reprod 2003;18:659–64.

34. Courbiere B, Oborski V, Braunstein D, Desparoir A, Noizet A, Gamerre M. Obstetric outcome of women with in vitro fertilization pregnancies hospitalized for ovarian hyperstimulation syndrome: a case-control study. Fertil Steril 2011;95:1629–32.

35. Haas J,Yinon Y, Meridor K, Hershko-Klement A, Orvieto R, Schiff E, et al. Is severe ovarian hyperstimulation syndrome associated with adverse pregnancy outcome? Evidence from a large case-control study. Am J Obstet Gynecol 2014; 210 Suppl 1: S329–30.

36. Mathur RS, Jenkins JM. Is ovarian hyperstimulation syndrome associated with a poor obstetric outcome? BJOG 2000;107:943–6.

37. Papanikolaou EG, Tournaye H, Verpoest W, Camus M, VernaeveV, Van Steirteghem A, et al. Early and late ovarian hyperstimulation syndrome:early pregnancy outcome and profile. Hum Reprod 2005;20:636–41.

38. CO Nastri, DM Teixeira, RM Moroni, VM Leitao, and WP Martins, "Ovarian hyperstimulation syndrome: pathophysiology, staging, prediction and prevention," Ultrasound in Obstetrics & Gynecology, 2015;45(4):377–393.

39. SR Soares, R Gómez, C Simón, JA García-Velasco, and A Pellicer, "Targeting the vascular endothelial growth factor system to prevent ovarian hyperstimulation syndrome," Human Reproduction Update, 2008;14(4):321–333.

40. TH Wang, SG Horng, CL Chang, et al. "Human chorionic gonadotropin-induced ovarian hyperstimulation syndrome is associated with up-regulation of vascular endothelial growth factor," Journal of Clinical Endocrinology and Metabolism, 2002;87(7):3300–3308.

41. C Gnoth, AN Schuring, K Friol, J Tigges, P Mallmann, and E Godehardt, "Relevance of anti-Mullerian hormone measurement in a routine IVF program," Human Reproduction, 2008;23 (6):1359–1365.

42. SL Broer, M Dólleman, BC Opmeer, BC Fauser, BW Mol, and FJM Broekmans, "AMH and AFC as predictors of excessive response in controlled ovarian hyperstimulation: a meta-analysis," Human Reproduction Update, 2011;17(1):46–54.

43. P Ocal, S Sahmay, M Cetin, T Irez, O Guralp, and I Cepni, "Serum anti-Müllerian hormone and antral follicle count as predictive markers of OHSS in ART cycles," Journal of Assisted Reproduction and Genetics, 2011;28(12):1197–1203.

44. EG Papanikolaou, C Pozzobon, EM Kolibianakis et al., "Incidence and prediction of ovarian hyperstimulation syndrome in women undergoing gonadotropin-releasing hormone antagonist in vitro fertilization cycles," Fertility and Sterility, 2006;85(1):112–120.

45. BK Tan and R Mathur, "Management of ovarian hyperstimulation syndrome. Produced on behalf of the BFS policy and practice committee," Human Fertility, 2013;16(3):151–159.

46. Joint SOGC-CFAS Clinical Practice Guideline, "The diagnosis and management of ovarian hyperstimulation syndrome," Journal of Obstetrics and Gynaecology Canada, 2011; 2068:1156–1162.

47. S Christin-Maitre, JN Hugues, and Recombinant FSH Study Group, "A comparative randomized multicentric study comparing the step-up versus step-down protocol in polycystic ovary syndrome," Human Reproduction, 2003; 18(8):1626–1631.

48. R Homburg, T Levy, and Z Ben-Rafael, "A comparative prospective study of conventional regimen with chronic low-dose administration of follicle-stimulating hormone for anovulation associated with polycystic ovary syndrome," Fertility and Sterility, 1995;63(4):729–733.

49. EM Elia, R Quintana, C Carrere et al., "Metformin decreases the incidence of ovarian hyperstimulation syndrome: an experimental study," Journal of Ovarian Research, 2013;6(1), article 62.

50. LO Tso, MF Costello, LE Albuquerque, RB Andriolo, and CR Macedo, "Metformin treatment before and during IVF or ICSI in women with polycystic ovary syndrome," Cochrane Database of Systematic Reviews, 2014;11:Article ID Cd006105.

51. S Palomba, A Falbo, and GB la Sala, "Effects of metformin in women with polycystic ovary syndrome treated with gonadotrophins for in vitro fertilisation and intracytoplasmic sperm injection cycles: a systematic review and meta-analysis of randomised controlled trials," BJOG: An International Journal of Obstetrics and Gynaecology, 2013;120(3):267–276.

52. Y El-Faissal, "Approaches to complete prevention of OHSS," Middle East Fertility Society Journal, 2014;19(1):13–15.

53. MF Costello, M Chapman, and U Conway, "A systematic review and meta-analysis of randomized controlled trials on metformin co-administration during gonadotrophin ovulation induction or IVF in women with polycystic ovary syndrome," Human Reproduction, 2006;21 (6):1387–1399.

54. A Delvigne and S Rozenberg, "A qualitative systematic review of coasting, a procedure to avoid ovarian hyperstimulation syndrome in IVF patients," Human Reproduction Update, 2002; 8(3):91–296.

55. P Devroey and P Adriaensen, "OHSS free clinic", facts, views and vision in ObGyn, 2011;3(1):43–45.

56. R Mathur and W Sumaya, "Prevention and management of ovarian hyperstimulation syndrome," Obstetrics, Gynaecology and Reproductive Medicine, 2008;18(1):18–22.

57. JG Schenker and D Weinstein, "Ovarian hyperstimulation syndrome: a current survey", Fertility and Sterility, 1978;30(3), 255–268.

Role of Lifestyle and Diet in PCOS

Savita Rani Singhal, Vandana Rani

Polycystic ovary syndrome (PCOS) is the commonest endocrine disorder in women of reproductive age group. It is a syndrome which includes manifestations due to anovulation (oligomenorrhea, other menstrual irregularities, infertility) and hyperandrogenism (hirsutism, oily skin, acne).

Two other components of PCOS are insulin resistance and obesity. Insulin resistance and obesity are present in 50–70% and 50–60% of patients with PCOS respectively.[1] Obese women with PCOS are at increased risk of anovulation and further infertility when compared to lean women with PCOS.[2] Obesity in women with PCOS has also been associated with reduced response to infertility treatments. Obese women are also more likely to suffer from obstetric complications like increased risk of spontaneous abortions and preterm labor, increased incidence of gestational diabetes mellitus, gestational hypertension, increased operative interferences, wound infections and thromboembolism. Thus, obese women with PCOS should be encouraged for weight loss before treatment of infertility.

Treatment protocols for PCOS aims at normalizing hyperandrogenism, restoring ovulation and improving the reproductive outcomes. It includes combination of oral contraceptives for managing menstrual irregularities, anti-androgens for hyperandrogenism, laparoscopic ovarian drilling, and ovulation inducing agents for infertility. Modifications in lifestyle of PCOS women are introduced to help in weight loss and further reduce insulin resistance in these women.

LIFESTYLE MODIFICATION (LSM) PROGRAMS

Lifestyle modifications refer to a combination of diet with exercise. Execution of new lifestyle could be enhanced by counseling sessions, psychological support and pharmacological adjuvant therapy.

The aim of LSM programs is to achieve and further maintain ideal healthy body weight. Small to moderate weight loss of about 5–10% is considered as significant in reducing insulin resistance and androgen levels. This further helps to restore ovulation, improve menstrual regularity, reduce the long-term risks of PCOS like cardiovascular disease, diabetes mellitus and thus, improves the quality of life. So, the lifestyle modification programs targeting weight loss (in obese women with PCOS) and prevention of weight gain (in lean women with PCOS) should be the first-line therapy in management of PCOS for prevention of long-term consequences.

Main challenge of LSM programs is maintenance of healthy dietary habits and physical activity attitudes for longer duration of time, but this could be achieved by behavioral therapy.

Components of LSM Programs

 I. Diet

 II. Exercise

III. Behavioral and cognitive approaches

I. Diet

The key strategy of diet in PCOS women is the negative energy balance. Several studies comparing the effects of two hypocaloric diets (energy deficit of 500 kcal/day) showed that the negative energy balance resulted in successful weight loss (4%), decreased dehydroepiandrosterone sulfate (DHEAS), decreased testosterone, increased SHBG concentrations and further amelioration of menstrual dysfunction and hirsutism.[3,4]

Thus, negative energy balance (around 350–1000 kcal/day) is an important factor leading to body weight and fat loss and further, improving insulin sensitivity and menstrual irregularities in PCOS women.

Dietary Components

Depending upon individual's dietary habits, preferences and metabolic goals, any range of dietary carbohydrates is accepted. There is no optimum amount of carbohydrate intake in diet for PCOS women. This has been proved as no significant differences in glucose or energy metabolism have been found with moderately low carbohydrate diets in two clinical trials.[5,6] Also, there is no dietary macronutrients or dietary pattern for PCOS.

In spite of the above facts, following points should be considered in the diet plans of the women with PCOS aiming at weight loss.

1. Always avoid a high carbohydrate breakfast.
2. Majority of carbohydrates should be consumed in the lunch time or if it is not possible then, there should be equal distribution of carbohydrate content in meals throughout the day.
3. Foods with low glycemic index should be included in the diet like 100% whole grains, oats, brown rice, sprouted grains, lettuce, green leafy vegetables, broccoli, spinach, green beans, chia seeds, flax seeds, citrus fruits, apple, soyabeans, etc.
4. Avoid excessive caffeine consumption, alcohol and smoking.
5. No recommendations are there for amount of protein in diet, however, addition of around 7–15 grams of protein in diet of PCOS women may offer some additional health benefits like lower postprandial glucose fluctuations and improvement in insulin sensitivity. This has been concluded from a meta-analysis of RCTs which suggested that high protein-low carbohydrate diets (within 6 months) may have some beneficial effects on weight loss in women with impaired glucose metabolism,[7] probably due to increased protein bound thermogenesis, increased satiety, possibly due to enhanced cholecystokinin production.[8,9] Moreover, many studies also concluded that dietary protein did not have any important effects on glucose metabolism and no differences were found between high and low protein diets.[5,6,10]
6. Dietary approaches to stop hypertension (DASH) diet is a low glycemic index, low energy density, high fiber and high complex carbohydrate diet (18% protein, 52% carbohydrate, 30% fat). Adherence to DASH eating patterns for 12 weeks had been shown to have beneficial effects on weight loss, SHBG, serum AMH and insulin metabolism in women with PCOS.[11] Women with PCOS should be encouraged for adoption of healthy dietary patterns such as DASH or Mediterranean style diet. These type of diets have high fiber and have antioxidant/anti-inflammatory nutrients which will add antidiabetic, antihyperlipidemic and antihypertensive properties to the diet.
7. Frequency and timing of meals is also an important component of diet plan in PCOS women. Six meal pattern is reported to have a beneficial effect on insulin sensitivity and reduction in subjective hunger in women with PCOS as compared to three meal pattern.[12] There may be a beneficial effect of increased meal frequency on body weight and glycemic control which may be attributed to:
   - Nutrient load spreading
   - Hunger reduction

- Lower levels of postprandial insulin
- Glucose uptake suppression (may be due to inhibitory effects of free fatty acids)
- Increased glucose clearance from the circulation

Thus, women with PCOS should be advised to increase the frequency of their meals and also, adhere to regular timing of the meals to ensure a gradual weight loss and to maintain a healthy weight for a longer duration of time.

8. Supplementation of vitamin D and micro-nutrients (folate, zinc, selenium) in PCOS women has not yet been recommended because there is still a great need for well-designed, long term, with adequate sample size clinical trials in women with PCOS.

ESHRE 2008 recommends any hypo-caloric diet (with a 500 kcal/day deficit) with reduced glycemic load with which patients can comply and achieve a 5% weight loss.[13]

Food pyramids have been designed to provide dietary guidance to the people and also emphasized the importance of eating a balanced, varied diet. Foods near the base of pyramid are categorized as 'good' foods and can be taken freely. Similarly, foods near the tip of pyramid are 'bad' and should be limited or avoided. Women with PCOS should also be taught about the food pyramid to help them to manage their balanced diet to ease their weight loss strategies.

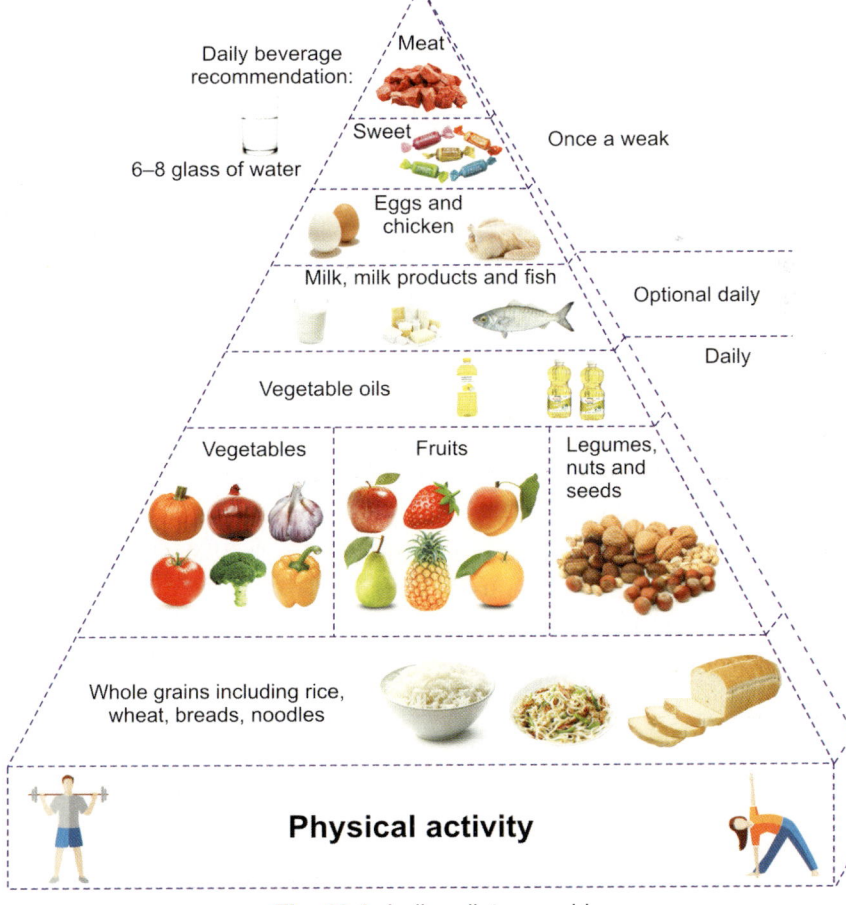

Daily beverage recommendation:

6–8 glass of water

Meat

Sweet — Once a weak

Eggs and chicken

Milk, milk products and fish — Optional daily

Vegetable oils — Daily

Vegetables   Fruits   Legumes, nuts and seeds

Whole grains including rice, wheat, breads, noodles

Physical activity

Fig. 19.1: Indian diet pyramid

II. Exercise

Exercise with physical activity stays an important component of lifestyle modification programmes in women with PCOS.

Regular physical exercise should be encouraged and advised to all women with PCOS especially to the obese women, at least 3–5 times weekly. The type, duration and frequency of exercise depends upon personal attitude, personal limitations and health conditions. Two main types of exercises which can be executed in PCOS women are as follows:

1. *Aerobic exercises:* Moderate to high/ vigorous intensity aerobic exercises have been preferred as a treatment of PCOS.[14]

   Moderate intensity exercises are those which cause an increase in heart rate by 55–70%. These exercises include brisk walking (5–7 km/hr), walking uphill, cycling (8–15 km/hr), low impact aerobics, gymnastics, moderate dancing, etc.[15]

   Vigorous intensity exercises cause an increase in heart rate by 70–90%. These include race walking, jogging/running, mountain climbing, cycling (>16 km/hr, 10 mph), high impact aerobics, karate or similar, circuit weight training, vigorous dancing and aerobic machines, etc.[15]

   Aerobic exercises have been found to effectively reduce total and abdominal body fat leading to improved menstrual frequency, reduced serum testosterone concentrations and fasting plasma glucose levels, and improved insulin sensitivity.[14,16]

   Women with PCOS typically have abdominal obesity. Straight leg raising and upper torso raising exercises are very helpful for reducing lower and upper abdominal fat respectively (Fig. 19.2).

2. *Progressive resistance training (PRT):* PRT or strength training schedules may also prove beneficial for obese women with PCOS. Literature suggests that PRT protocol is associated with practice of calisthenics (exercises in which body's own

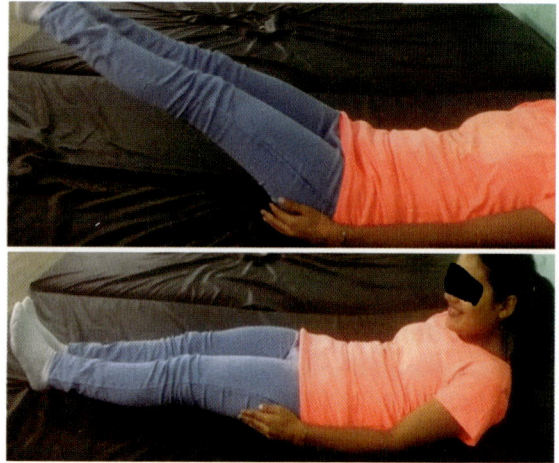

Fig. 19.2: Straight leg raising and upper torso raising exercises

weight is the primary tool). These exercises concomitantly cause increase in lean muscle mass and reduction in body fat.[17] Increase in lean muscle mass causes the body to increase its caloric expenditure and basal metabolic rate. The loss of body fat is probably mediated by increase in basal metabolic rate. This anabolic action adds to improved insulin sensitivity.[18] PRT also improves daily functional capacity and muscle strength of the individual.

A training schedule incorporating both aerobic exercises and PRT could prove beneficial in improvement of physical health in women with PCOS; thereby, improving the quality of life in these women.

Women should be counselled that various forms of physical exercises do not always require expensive gyms and fitness centers. Brisk/race walking, jogging, running, dancing, cycling, etc. are amongst the options which could be easily practiced in community centers or sports grounds with minimal equipment.

Yoga in PCOS Women

The holistic approaches in the management of PCOS are yoga and meditation. These approaches are helpful in dealing with the root causes of PCOS, i.e. obesity and stress.

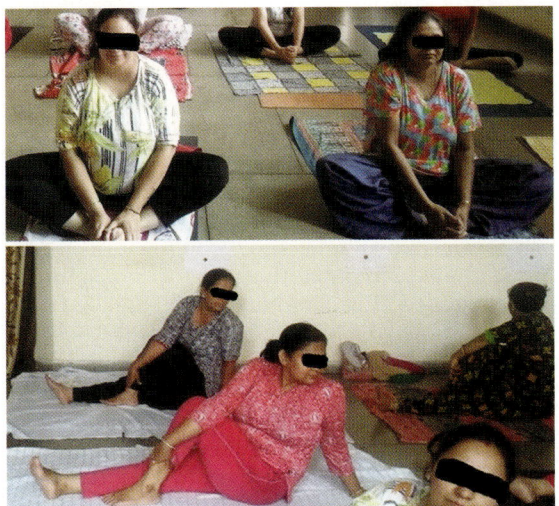

Fig. 19.3: Various yoga postures

Regular practice of various yoga postures (Fig. 19.3) for at least 30–60 minutes/day have been found to improve ovarian blood supply, helps in weight loss and ameliorates anxiety and depression in these patients. So, yoga should also be considered as a part of LSM programmes in the management of women suffering with PCOS.

Combination of aerobic and resistance training exercises for a period of at least 30 minutes/day can improve metabolic control and help in weight loss in obese PCOS women. Yoga is a traditional and spiritual way of overcoming the chronic stress, anxiety and depression in PCOS women and is of paramount importance in weight loss and for improving insulin resistance.

III. Behavioral and Cognitive Approaches

Behavioral therapy is also an important pillar of LSM programmes. Basic aim of behavioral therapy is to increase the psychological strength, stability of mind and ability to cope with everyday's stress. Patients should be counselled personally or in groups. Constant support and motivation is provided for weight loss and maintenance of balanced weight. Psychological factors such as anxiety and depressive symptoms, body image concerns and disordered eating should be considered to optimize healthy lifestyle engagement. All patient interactions should be patient-centered and patient's culture and ethnic background should be respected.

Motivational interviewing and established behavior techniques are more effective than traditional advice giving for changes in weight, diet or exercise. Women should be counseled about setting goals, techniques for achieving those goals, time management techniques, problem solving, self-monitoring and relapse prevention techniques. Women should be taught about slow eating techniques and they should also be told not to get distracted by television or any type of social media while eating meals. Counselling sessions of the women with PCOS also increase the degree of motivation for certain physical activities and promote better adherence to the training programmes. Family support in these patients also plays a great role in improvement of outcomes. Written or audio-visual resources can also be used during the counselling sessions. Thus, behavioral and psychological therapy in women with PCOS help in adoption of healthy lifestyle and were found to have beneficial effects on the well-being, health, and exercise behavior of PCOS women.

EXISTING GUIDELINES

Australian PCOS-alliance 2010 and the society of obstetricians and gynecologists of Canada (SOGC) recommend only lifestyle modification (diet and exercise) as first line therapy in women with PCOS for a duration of 3–6 months, not in combination with pharmacological ovulation inducing agents.[19, 20] Moreover, Australian PCOS-alliance 2010 recommends against the use of pharmacological ovulation inducing agents, until appropriate weight loss has been achieved in patients with BMI ≥35 kg/m². RCOG 2014 also recommend lifestyle modification as first line, but with preceding and/or accompanying pharmacological treatment.[21]

CONCLUSION

Life style modification programmes have nowadays become the key strategy in management of PCOS patients. Hypocaloric diet with physical activity play an important role in weight loss and maintenance of balanced weight. Yoga is also recommended as a part of LSM programmes. Above all, behavioral therapy approach is very important for motivation and adherence of women with PCOS to the LSM protocols.

REFERENCES

1. Goodarzi MO, Dumesic DA, Chazenbalk G, Azziz R, 2011 Polycystic ovary syndrome: etiology, pathogenesis and diagnosis. Nat Rev Endocrinol 7: 219–31.
2. Jamil AS, Alalaf SK, Al-Tawil NG, Al-Shawaf T. Comparison of clinical and hormonal characteristics among four phenotypes of polycystic ovary syndrome based on the Rotterdam criteria. Arch Gynecol Obstet 2016;293:447–56.
3. Mehrabani HH, Salehpour S, Amiri Z, Farahani SJ, Meyer BJ, Tahbaz F. Beneficial effects of a high-protein, low-glycemic-load hypocaloric diet in overweight and obese women with polycystic ovary syndrome: a randomized controlled intervention study. J Am Coll Nutr. 2012; 31(2): 117–25.
4. Marzouk TM, Sayed Ahmed WA. Effect of dietary weight loss on menstrual regularity in obese young adult women with polycystic ovary syndrome. *J Pediatr Adolesc Gynecol*. 2015; 28(6): 457–61.
5. Moran LJ, Noakes M, Clifton PM, Tomlinson L, Galletly C, Norman RJ. Dietary composition in restoring reproductive and metabolic physiology in overweight women with polycystic ovary syndrome. J Clin Endocrinol Metab. 2003; 88(2): 812–9.
6. Stamets K, Taylor DS, Kunselman A, Demers LM, Pelkman CL, Legro RS. A randomized trial of the effects of two types of short-term hypocaloric diets on weight loss in women with polycystic ovary syndrome. Fertil Steril. 2004; 81(3):630–7.
7. Dong JY, Zhang ZL, Wang PY, Qin LQ. Effects of high-protein diets on body weight, glycaemic control, blood lipids and blood pressure in type 2 diabetes: meta-analysis of randomised controlled trials. Br J Nutr. 2013;110(5):781–9.
8. Koppes LL, Boon N, Nooyens AC, van Mechelen W, Saris WH. Macronutrient distribution over a period of 23 years in relation to energy intake and body fatness. Br J Nutr. 2009;101(1):108–15.
9. de la Iglesia R, Loria-Kohen V, Zulet MA, Martinez JA, Reglero G, Ramirez de Molina A. Dietary strategies implicated in the prevention and treatment of metabolic syndrome. Int J Mol Sci. 2016;17(11):E1877.
10. Papakonstantinou E, Triantafillidou D, Panagiotakos DB, Iraklianou S, Berdanier CD, Zampelas A. A high protein low fat meal does not influence glucose and insulin responses in obese individuals with or without type 2 diabetes. J Hum Nutr Diet. 2010;23(2):183–9.
11. Foroozanfard F, Rafiei H, Samimi M, et al. The effects of dietary approaches to stop hypertension diet on weight loss, anti-Mullerian hormone and metabolic profiles in women with polycystic ovary syndrome: a randomized clinical trial. Clin Endocrinol (Oxf). 2017.
12. Papakonstantinou E, Kechribari I, Mitrou P, et al. Effect of meal frequency on glucose and insulin levels in women with polycystic ovary syndrome: a randomised trial. Eur J Clin Nutr. 2016;70(5):588–594.
13. Thessaloniki ESHRE/ASRM-Sponsored PCOS Consensus Workshop Group. Consensus on infertility treatment related to polycystic ovary syndrome. Hum Reprod 2008;23:462–77.
14. Thomson RL, Buckley JD, Noakes M, Clifton PM, Norman RJ, Brinkworth GD. The effect of a hypocaloric diet with and without exercise training on body composition, cardiometabolic risk profile, and reproductive function in overweight and obese women with polycystic ovary syndrome. J Clin Endocrinol Metab 2008;93(09):3373–3380.
15. Norton, K, L Norton, and D Sadgrove, Position statement on physical activity and exercise intensity terminology. Journal of Science and Medicine in Sport, 2010. 13(5): p. 496–502.

16. Harrison CL, Stepto NK, Hutchison SK, Teede HJ. The impact of intensified exercise training on insulin resistance and fitness in overweight and obese women with and without polycystic ovary syndrome. Clin Endocrinol (Oxf) 2012; 76(03):351–7.

17. Vizza L, Smith CA, Swaraj S, Agho K, Cheema BS. The feasibility of progressive resistance training in women with polycystic ovary syndrome: a pilot randomized controlled trial. BMC Sports Sci Med Rehabil 2016;8:14.

18. Tresierras MA, Balady GJ. Resistance training in the treatment of diabetes and obesity: mechanisms and outcomes. J Cardiopulm Rehabil Prev 2009;29(02):67–75.

19. Teede HJ, Misso ML, Deeks AA,Moran LJ, Stuckey BG,Wong JL, et al. Assessment and management of polycystic ovary syndrome: Summary of an evidence-based guideline. Med J Aust 2011;195:S65–112.

20. Vause TD, Cheung AP, Sierra S, Claman P, Graham J, Guillemin JA,et al. Ovulation induction in polycystic ovary syndrome. J Obstet Gynaecol Can 2010;32:495–502.

21. Long term consequences of polycystic ovary syndrome. RCOG.Green-top Guideline No. 33. Available from: https://www.rcog.org.uk/globalassets/documents/guidelines/gt33_longtermpcos.pdf. [Last accessed on2016 Sep 07].

Surgical Management of Polycystic Syndrome: Laparoscopic Ovarian Drilling

B Ramesh

INTRODUCTION

Polycystic ovary syndrome (PCOS) is a predominant cause of anovulatory infertility,[1] with prevalence rate of 17–20% (Rotterdam diagnostic criteria).[2,3]

PATHOPHYSIOLOGY

The three prevalent theories for the pathogenesis of PCOS are as follows:

1. Hypothalamic-pituitary dysfunction results in gonadotropin-releasing hormone and luteinizing hormone dysfunction, which then has downstream effects on ovarian hormone production.
2. A primary ovarian defect (with or without an adrenal defect) in steroidogenesis results in hyperandrogenism.
3. A metabolic disorder characterized by peripheral insulin resistance exerts adverse effects on the hypothalamus, pituitary, ovaries, and, possibly, the adrenal gland.

There are three sets of diagnostic criteria have been utilized for adult women, including the 1990 National Institutes of Child and Human Development criteria (which requires chronic oligoovulation with clinical or biochemical signs of hyperandrogenism), 2003 Rotterdam criteria (which requires two of three criteria—chronic oligoovulation or anovulation, clinical or biochemical signs of hyperandrogenism, and polycystic ovaries), 2006 the criteria of the Androgen Excess Society (which defines PCOS as hyperandrogenism manifested as hirsutism and hyper-androgenemia, and ovarian dysfunction based on chronic oligoovulation or anovulation and polycystic ovaries)[4,5] and 2012 National Institute of Health Workshop includes Endorsement of Rotterdam criteria, acknowledging its limitations, and suggesting the name PCOS should be changed. The prevalence of the disease has increased tremendously, and often medical treatment is not helpful in controlling the disease and improving fertility.

The key management strategy should be directed at altering lifestyle variables. Exercise regimens, particularly when coordinated with a group of similar women, have been shown to be beneficial. However, this approach should be part of all therapies for PCOS, acknowledging that some thin and normal-weight women with PCOS probably already have a healthy lifestyle.

ULTRASOUND FEATURES OF THE POLYCYSTIC OVARY

A typical polycystic ovary has following characteristic ultrasonographic appearance:

1. Enlarged ovaries that are usually more spherical in shape
2. Multiple small follicles of similar size arranged around the periphery, giving the appearance of a "string-of-pearls"
3. The increased and hyperechoic stroma occupying the center of the ovaries.
4. Higher intraovarian stromal blood flow. Among these features, follicle number and ovarian volume are the sonographic

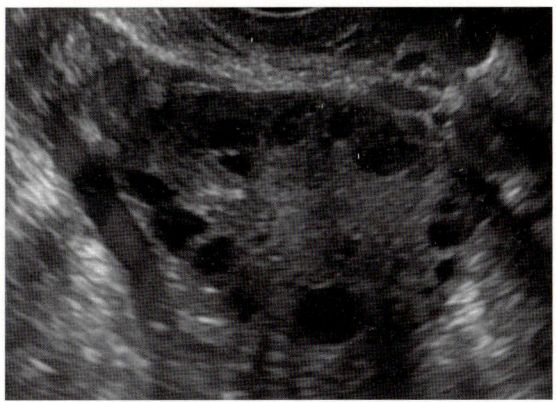

Fig. 20.1: Ultrasonogram of polycystic ovary showing the characteristic necklace pattern

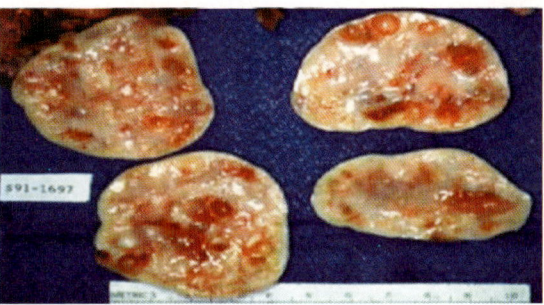

Fig. 20.2: Surgical specimen of polycystic ovaries

parameters chosen to establish the diagnostic criteria for polycystic ovary. Figure 20.1 shows various ultrasonographic features of polycystic ovary.

TREATMENT FOR WOMEN WITH POLYCYSTIC OVARY SYNDROME

The multiple treatment options available for the treatment of polycystic ovarian syndrome are summarized in Table 20.1.

Surgical Management

Surgical option of removal of ovarian tissue to improve the gonadotropins production has been in practice for a long time. In 1930s, surgical ovarian wedge resection was first performed via laparotomy. Three-fourths of each ovary was resected during the procedure and about 60% pregnancy rate was achieved. With the risk of postoperative adhesion formation, the procedure was later abandoned. Figure 20.2 shows cut section of surgically removed polycystic ovaries.

Laparoscopic ovarian drilling was first described by Gjonnaess in 1984.[6] Increased incidence of failure of medical management of infertility associated with polycystic ovarian syndrome and advances in minimal access surgery made the concept of ovarian drilling appealingly high.

Indications

The main indication for laparoscopic ovarian drilling is clomiphene resistant PCOS with associated infertility.[7–10] Other indications include severe PCOS, hyperandrogenic stroma, and repeated abortions.

Mechanism of Action

The exact mechanism is yet to be elucidated. The most plausible one is the destruction of ovarian follicles and stroma resulting in a decrease in androgen and inhibin levels and a secondary rise in follicle-stimulating hormone

Table 20.1: Common complaints and treatment options in polycystic ovarian syndrome	
Complaint	*Treatment options*
Infertility	Letrozole, clomiphene, with or without metformin, gonadotropins, ovarian cautery ("drilling")
Skin manifestations	Oral contraceptive + antiandrogen (spironolactone, finasteride), GnRH agonists
Abnormal bleeding	Cyclic progestogen, oral contraceptives
Weight, metabolic concerns	Diet/lifestyle management, metformin

(FSH) levels.[11–13] Laparoscopic ovarian drilling may also increase ovarian blood flow and postsurgical local growth factors. An improvement of insulin sensitivity after laparoscopic ovarian drilling has also been suggested as one mechanism.

Procedure

Basic requirements: Laparoscopic ovarian drilling is a simple procedure and can be performed in any operation theatre with general anesthesia. It also simultaneously allows for complete inspection of the abdomen for diagnostic evaluation for infertility like endometriosis, pelvic inflammatory disease (Fig. 20.3). It allows multiple ovarian biopsies, multi-perforation by monopolar electro-coagulation. Apart from basics of laparoscopy, the procedure is relatively easy to master.

Ovarian Drilling

After the initial laparoscopic instruments are inserted, the abdomen is inspected for any pelvic pathologies (Fig. 20.2). This is an essential step and should not be overlooked, since direct examination under laparoscopy is the most sensitive modality to pick up abnormalities that are often missed during routine evaluation for infertility.

The ovary is immobilized with laparoscopic forceps and the treatment is performed using the needle electrode on both ovaries. The needle is inserted as perpendicularly as possible to the ovarian surface and stroma. The whole length of the needle (8 mm) (Fig. 20.3) is inserted into the ovary, and it is activated with 40 watts of coagulating current for 2 seconds at each point. Figure 20.5 shows the unipolar electrocautery used for the procedure. Release of fluid from the underlying "follicles" is usually seen with each puncture (Fig. 20.6). During the procedure, it is important to hold the ovary away from the bowel and other vital structures to avoid potential sparking and arcing from electrical current. Care must be taken to avoid the hilum of the ovary and the ovarian blood supply (Fig. 20.4). At the completion of the procedure, suction and irrigation is done in the peritoneal cavity (Fig. 20.7). Figures 20.8

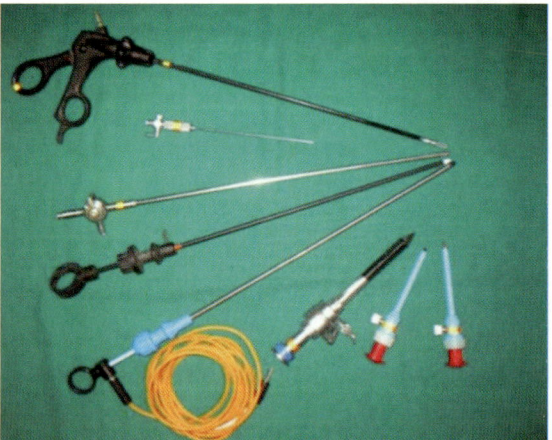

Fig. 20.4: Instruments used in laparoscopic drilling

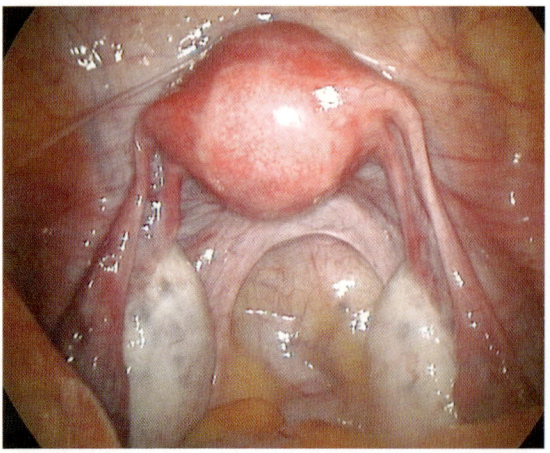

Fig. 20.3: Laparoscopic pelvic view of the bilateral polycystic ovaries. Note the multiple dark discoloration on the surface of each ovary; these are ovarian follicles that are chosen for drilling

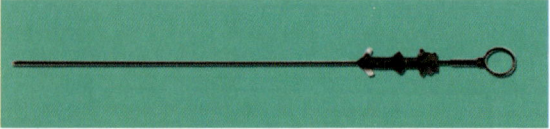

Fig. 20.5: Unipolar electrode used for electrocautery

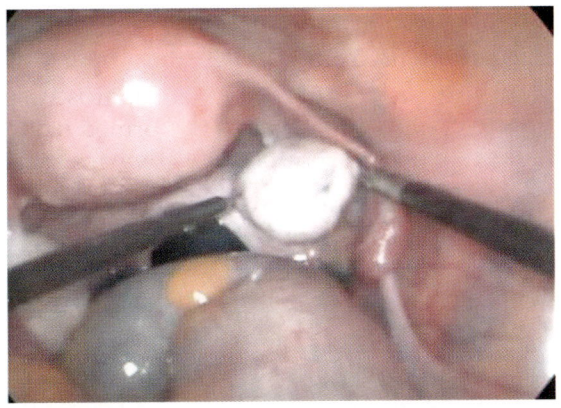

Fig. 20.6: Immobilization of ovaries with laparoscopic forceps

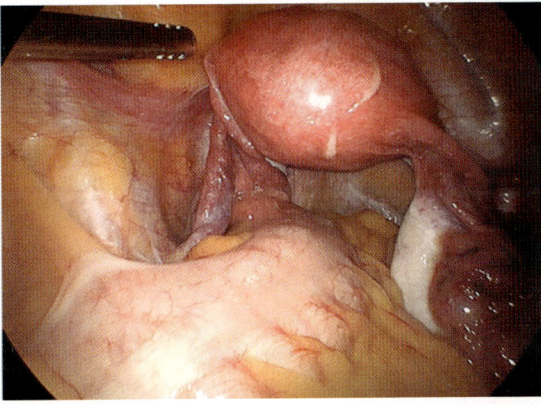

Fig. 20.9: Suction and irrigation in laparoscopic ovarian drilling with suction cannula

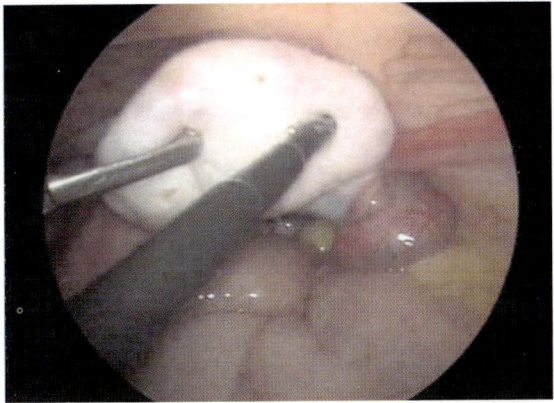

Fig. 20.7: Ovarian drilling done with a unipolar electrode. Note the direct application of electrocautery over the ovarian surface

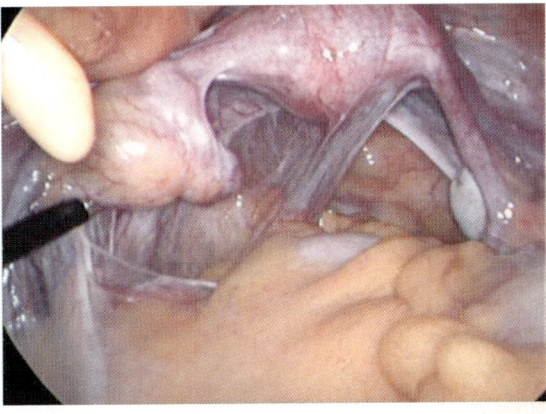

Fig. 20.10: Postoperative pelvic adhesions following laparoscopic ovarian drilling

to 20.10 show laparoscopic ovarian drilling being carried out.

Reproductive and Endocrinal Changes after Laparoscopic Ovarian Drilling

The ovarian drilling subsequently causes decline in the serum levels of androgens, inhibin and LH and an increase in FSH levels. The subsequent correction of the ovarian-pituitary feedback mechanism will lead to follicular recruitment, maturation and ovulation. Other procedures including multiple ovarian punch biopsy are less popular. The spontaneous ovulation and pregnancy rates after various techniques of laparoscopic ovarian drilling, which have

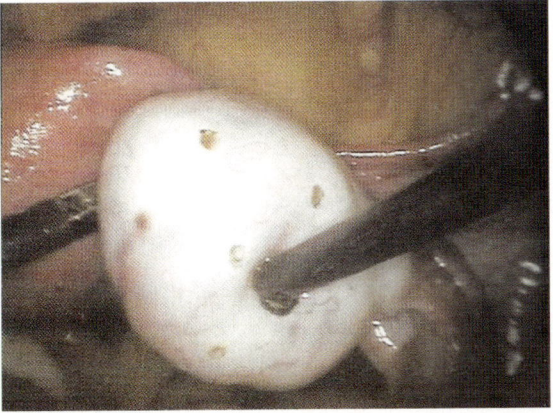

Fig. 20.8: Multiple drill holes seen over the ovarian surface. The ovary is being drilled further

varied from 30–90% to 13–88% respectively, within 1 year of the procedure.

Complications of Surgery

Intraoperative complications mainly involve complications of laparoscopy or general anesthesia. There is also a risk of an electrical accident to the adjacent organs when using monopolar current. There is additional risk of bleeding and injury to iliac veins.

In case of postoperative complications, periadnexal adhesions are a constant issue. Theoretically, such adhesions could cause infertility and pelvic pain, but no study has established a clear link between adhesion and infertility. Ovarian wedge resection has been abandoned because it led to pelvic adhesions in almost 100% of cases, but these adhesions were not associated with infertility. The risk of damaging the ovarian reserve, i.e. destroying part of the surface of the ovary may risk eliminating not only the excess tissue producing androgens but also the vital ovarian follicles. Loss of these follicles could damage the ovarian reserve and make the patient less fertile.

Modifications of the Procedure

Several lasers including carbon dioxide (CO_2), Argon, KTP, and Nd:YAG laser have also been used for laparoscopic treatment of PCOS. The use of the CO_2 laser is associated with smoke production that might obscure the view and require to be evacuated intermittently. Argon and KTP lasers are associated with less smoke production and allow for deeper penetration. Contrary to other lasers, the Nd:YAG laser can be delivered using a flexible fibre delivery system equipped with sapphire tips. The results of laser surgery for PCOS are inferior to those of electrocautery.

Predictors of Success

On an average, 15–30% of anovulatory PCOS women fail to respond to laparoscopic ovarian drilling, because of inadequate destruction of ovarian stroma or resistance of the ovaries. The rationality of increasing the number of punctures or thermal energy applied to improve response at the high risks of adhesions and premature ovarian failure (POF).

Pregnancy Outcomes after Laparoscopic Ovarian Drilling

Multiple pregnancy rate varies from 1% to 10%, but it is lower than gonadotropins, thus making laparoscopic ovarian drilling an attractive option for clomiphene citrate-resistant PCOS. Laparoscopic ovarian drilling does not seem to be associated with risk of gestational diabetes mellitus.

Cost-effectiveness

One course of gonadotropin therapy results in a single ovulatory cycle with the need for intensive monitoring. Laparoscopic ovarian drilling on the other hand is more cost-effective, as a single-treatment results in several mono-ovulatory cycles thus making possible multiple attempts at conception. Although iatrogenic adhesion formation and decreased ovarian reserve are potential complications in laparoscopic ovarian drilling they can be minimized by limiting the number of punctures and energy applied.

CONCLUSION

In summary, laparoscopic ovarian drilling is the treatment of choice in anovuatory clomiphene resistant polycystic ovarian syndrome as it is associated with a lower risk of multiple pregnancy and ovarian hyper-stimulation syndrome. Nevertheless, laparoscopic ovarian drilling carries risks such as pelvic infection, postoperative adhesion formation, risks of general anesthesia and the theoretical risk of premature ovarian failure. All these should be taken into consideration before embarking on this procedure. Careful selection and counseling of patients is very important along with a skilled laparoscopic surgeon.

REFERENCES

1. Overbeek A, Lambalk CB. Phenotypic and pharmacogenetic aspects of ovulation induction in WHO II anovulatory women. Gynecol Endocrinol 2009;25:222–34.

2. March WA, Moore VM, Willson KJ, Phillips DI, Norman RJ, Davies MJ. The prevalence of polycystic ovary syndrome in a community sample assessed under contrasting diagnostic criteria. Hum Reprod 2010;25:544–51.

3. Yildiz BO, Bozdag G, Yapici Z, Esinler I, Yarali H. Prevalence, phenotype and cardiometabolic risk of polycystic ovary syndrome under different diagnostic criteria. Hum Reprod 2012;27: 3067–73.

4. Norman RJ, Dewailly D, Legro RS, Hickey TE. Polycystic ovary syndrome. Lancet 2007;370: 685–97.

5. Yii MF, Lim CE, Luo X, Wong WS, Cheng NC, Zhan X. Polycystic ovarian syndrome in adolescence. Gynecol Endocrinol 2009;25:634–9.

6. Gjonnaess H. Polycystic ovarian syndrome treated by ovarian electrocautery through the laparoscope. Fertil Steril 1984;41:20–5.

7. Abu Hashim H. Clomiphene citrate alternatives for the initial management of polycystic ovary syndrome: an evidence-based approach. Arch Gynecol Obstet 2012;285:1737–45.

8. Smithson DS, Vause TDR, Cheung AP. No. 362- Ovulation Induction in Polycystic Ovary Syndrome. J Obstet Gynaecol Can 2018;40:978–87.

9. Abu Hashim H, Al-Inany H, De Vos M, Tournaye H. Three decades after Gjonnaess's laparoscopic ovarian drilling for treatment of PCOS; what do we know? An evidence-based approach. Arch Gynecol Obstet 2013;288:409–22.

10. Fernandez H, Morin-Surruca M, Torre A, Faivre E, Deffieux X, Gervaise A. Ovarian drilling for surgical treatment of polycystic ovarian syndrome: a comprehensive review. Reprod Biomed Online 2011;22:556–68.

11. Flyckt RL, Goldberg JM. Laparoscopic ovarian drilling for clomiphene-resistant polycystic ovary syndrome. Semin Reprod Med 2011; 29:138–46.

12. Felemban A, Tan SL, Tulandi T. Laparoscopic treatment of polycystic ovaries with insulated needle cautery: a reappraisal. Fertil Steril 2000; 73:266–9.

13. Kato M, Kikuchi I, Shimaniki H, et al. Efficacy of laparoscopic ovarian drilling for polycystic ovary syndrome resistant to clomiphene citrate. J Obstet Gynaecol Res 2007;33:174–80.

Bariatric Surgery and PCOS

Shashwat Jani, Tapan Shah

INTRODUCTION

Obesity is a major health problem in this era, which gives you many accompanying projects like diabetes, hypertension, cardiovascular diseases, stroke, etc. Bariatric surgery or say weight-loss surgery has been very much accepted in last decade and has undergone various research for the more and more procedures. It has been recently recognised that weight reduction surgery modifies the metabolic and hormonal states too which are associated with comorbidities.[1,2]

POLYCYSTIC OVARIAN SYNDROME[3,4]

It is not just a syndrome, but it is a cluster of diseases which are acquired due to imbalance in the hormonal structure of the female genital system.

In polycystic ovarian disease, ovaries become polycystic when they are stimulated to generate more and more amounts of androgen hormones specifically testosterone. Fig. 21.1 summarizes the pathophysiology of PCOS.

In combination with mostly genetic susceptibility, the other causes may be any of the following:

1. The anterior pituitary gland secretes excessive luteinizing hormone (LH) or
2. Hyperinsulinemia

If we see some brief about PCOS or PCOD, its most accepted name is due to its presentation on sonography examination of poly (multiple) cysts in the ovaries. They (cysts) are

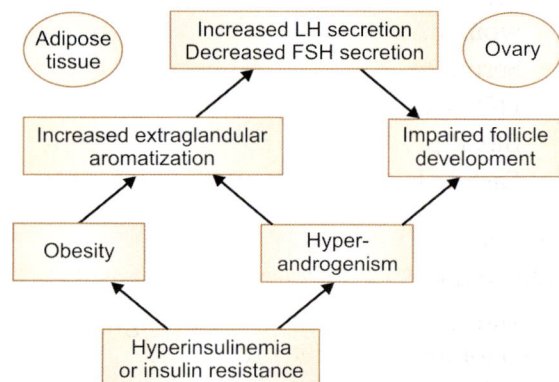

Fig. 21.1: Depicting pathophysiology of PCOS[3–5]

immature follicles in realty. The development of the follicles have stopped at an early antral stage due to ovarian dysfunction or arrested function.[3, 4]

PCOS → Increased frequency of hypothalamic GnRH pulses → Increase LH/FSH ratio

PCOS is associated with some of the deadliest condition which should be considered in the treatment protocols:

1. Insulin resistance or hyperinsulinemia
2. Obesity
3. Hypertension
4. Dyslipidemia
5. Sleep apnea
6. Metabolic syndrome

WHAT IS METABOLIC SYNDROME?[3–8]

We are focusing more here on the metabolic syndrome and association with PCOS.

Metabolic syndrome is a cluster of conditions:

1. Increased blood pressure
2. High blood sugar
3. Excess body fat around waist
4. Abnormal cholesterol or triglyceride levels

These all together increase the risk of the heart disease, stroke and diabetes.

Criteria for the Metabolic Syndrome

- Waist circumference 88 cm or more in women.
- Serum triglyceride 150 mg/dL or above
- HDL cholesterol 50 mg/dL or low
- Blood pressure 130/85 mm Hg or more
- Fasting blood glucose 110 mg/dL or more

Relation of PCOS and Metabolic Syndrome[5–9]

Patients with PCOS are at high risk of developing metabolic syndrome.

33% of the patients with PCOS have metabolic syndrome.

Most patients with PCOS and metabolic syndrome are over-weight or say obese and so they are at risk of cardiovascular diseases.

On the other hand if we will see frequency of obesity is 30–70% in the women with PCOS, which will give them anovulation-infertility also.

(5% weight loss even will restore ovulation by 50–60%).

Bariatric Surgery and its Role in PCOS[1–6]

As we saw in previous some pages that polycystic ovarian syndrome is associated with hormonal imbalance and due to that there are morbidities like diabetes mellitus, obesity, and due to obesity patient can get cardiovascular diseases, stroke, infertility (due to anovulation).

So to decrease morbidity and ultimately improve lifestyle of the patient she needs to decrease weight and hence she needs either diet modification or some weight-loss surgery.

Bariatric surgery is currently the most effective method to treat morbid obesity. Excess weight is the weight above the patient's ideal body weight.

Obesity is defined as body mass index (BMI) and excess body weight. Table 21.1 elaborates on classification of BMI.

Bariatric procedures are described according to their mechanism of weight loss:

1. Restrictive (vertical sleeve gastrectomy, lap assisted gastric banding)
2. Malabsorptive (biliopancreatic diversion, duodenal switch)
3. Combination of restrictive and malabsorptive

Here we will discuss about most common four procedures done for weight loss effectively.

1. Duodenal switch/BPD
2. Gastric bypass
3. Sleeve gastrectomy
4. Adjustable gastric banding

TABLE 21.1: Definition of obesity according to BMI and excess body weight

Category		BMI	% over ideal body weight
Underweight		<18.5	
Normal		18.5–24.9	
Overweight		25.0–29.9	
Obesity	(Class 1)	30–34.9	>20%
Severe obesity	(Class 2)	35–39.9	>100%
	(Class 3)	40–49.9	
Super obesity		>50	>250%

It is a surgical procedure (Fig. 21.2) in which the stomach is divided into 2 parts—a small upper pouch and a larger lower "remnant" pouch and then the small intestine is anastomosed to both.

Physiology behind the gastric bypass is that it reduces the size of the stomach by 90%. A normal stomach can stretch, sometimes up to 1L, while the pouch of the gastric bypass may be approximately 15 mL in size. The gastric bypass pouch is usually formed from the part of the stomach which can be stretched least. Over the time, the size of the connection between the stomach and intestine and the ability of the small intestine to hold a greater volume of food.

When the patient takes a small amount of food, the first response is a stretching of the wall of the stomach pouch, stimulating nerves which tell the brain that the stomach is full. The patient feels a sensation of fullness, as if they had just eaten a large meal—but with just a thumb-full of food.

Here (Fig. 21.3) stomach is reduced to 15% of its normal size, by surgical removal of a portion at the side of the greater curvature. The result gives a sleeve or tube like structure.

In vertical sleeve gastrectomy, longitudinal resection of the stomach is done from antrum to cardia.

The band is placed at the upper part of the stomach which creates a very small pouch which can hold hardly half cup of the food (Fig. 21.4). As the pouch fills with food, and the band slows the passage of food from the pouch to the lower part of the stomach, patient will feel full.

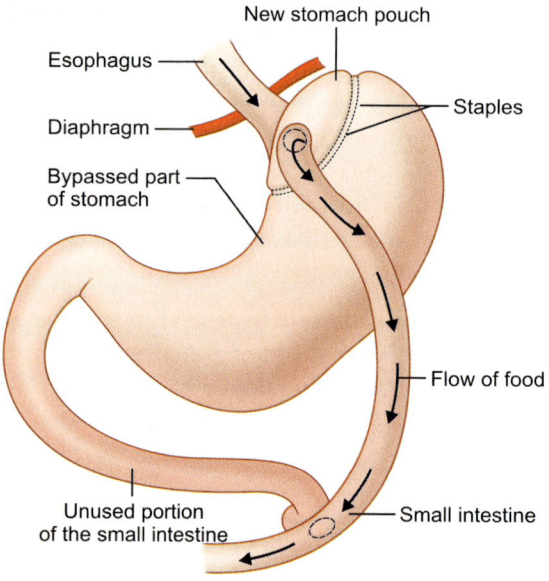

Fig. 21.2: Roux En-Y gastric bypass surgery

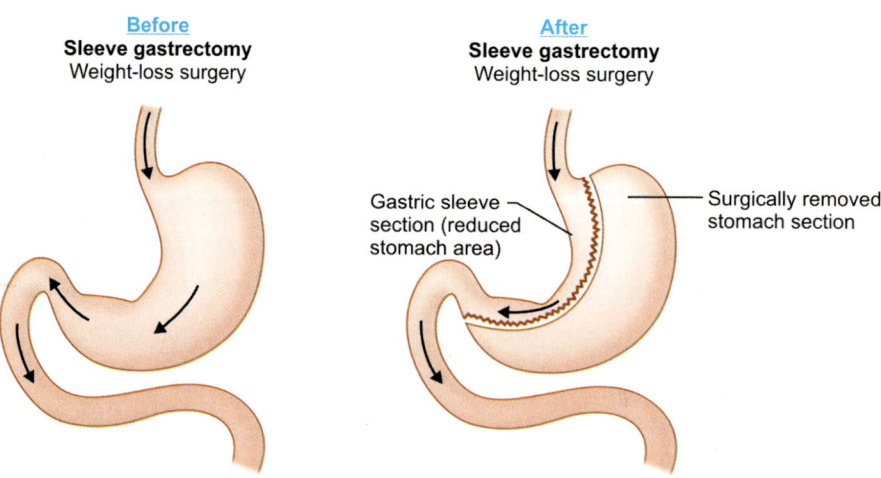

Fig. 21.3: Vertical sleeve gastrectomy

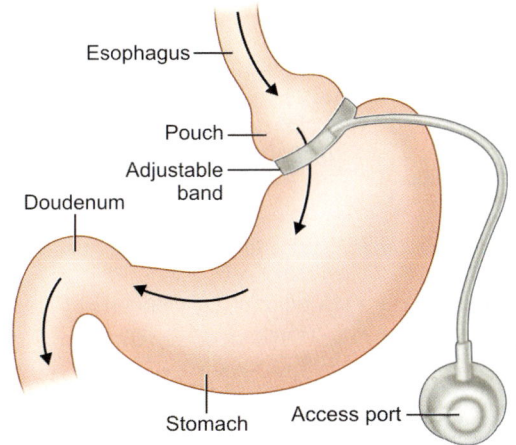

Fig 21.4: Laparoscopic assisted gastric banding

The band is an inflatable silicone device. Band is inflated with the saline with capacity of 4 to 15 mL. The band is kept not so loose not so tight.

Biliopancreatic diversion or the pancreatic switch includes the following steps:

Step 1: Subtotal gastrectomy leaving a proximal 200–300 ml pouch.

Step 2: The small bowel is divided 250 cm from the IC junction and a common channel is formed by completing the Roux En-Y enteroenterostomy around 50–60 cm from IC junction. Roux limb is anastomosed with the gastric pouch.

In the duodenal switch sleeve gastrectomy along the lesser curvature of the stomach leaves the antrum, pylorus and the first portion of the duodenum in continuity (Fig. 21.5). Here duodenoileostomy is made using 250 cm alimentary limb and than enteroenterostomy is done.

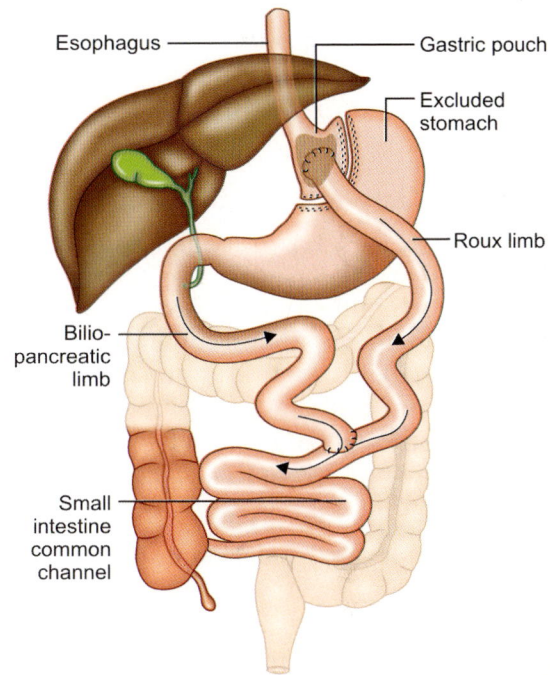

Fig. 21.5: Biliopancreatic diversion/duodenal switch

TABLE 21.2: Pros and cons of the all four types of procedure[1, 2]

Surgery	Pros	Cons
Gastric bypass surgery	• Most successful • Two-thirds of excess body weight loss in 1.5–2 years	• Nutritional deficiency (vitamin B_{12}/folic acid) • Dumping syndrome
Laparoscopic gastric banding	• Simple surgery • Easy to loose or tight the band post-surgery • Early weight loss post-tightening the band • Postsurgery complication rate is low • Loose half of excess body weight in 1.5–2 years	• More follow ups • Need to change the band if leaking • Slippage of the band • Nausea/vomiting/GERD/difficulty in swallowing • Increased risk of gallstones

(contd.)

TABLE 21.2: Pros and cons of the all four types of procedure[1,2] (contd.)

Surgery	Pros	Cons
Vertical sleeve gastrectomy	• Less complex than gastric bypass • Better controlling hunger than lap banding • Less time for surgery (30–60 minutes) • Less complications	• Nutritional deficiency • Weight loss is slower as compared to gastric bypass

BPD/duodenal switch	• Most helpful for morbid obese patients
	• Good if other surgeries not helpful
	• Gives highest rate of weight loss
		• High rate of complications related to surgery
		• Nutritional deficiencies
		  Calcium
		  Iron
		  Fat soluble vitamins
		• Protein energy malabsorbtion

Emerging Techniques in Bariatric Surgery[12,13]

Bariatric surgery has travelled to the new horizons in the last decade from open surgeries to multiport laparoscopic surgeries to single incision laparoscopic surgery to natural orifice transluminal endoscopic surgery (NOTES):

1. Intragastric balloons
2. Endoluminal vertical gastroplasty
3. Transoral gastroplasty
4. Endoscopic duodenal jejunal sleeve

Intragastric Balloons[12]

They are older methods with fewer devices where balloons are kept through endoscopy into the stomach under vision with help of endoscope and inflated with 500–600 mL of saline. To remove the balloon they are deflated with needles or endoscopic snares. Figure 21.6 shows intragastric balloons.

Endoluminal Vertical Gastroplasty

Here plication of gastroesophageal junction is done with device endoclinch. Because of the suture line distention of the stomach is restricted.

Transoral Gastroplasty[12,13]

In this technique, endoscopic stapplers with do full thickness plication of the proximal stomach (Fig. 21.7).

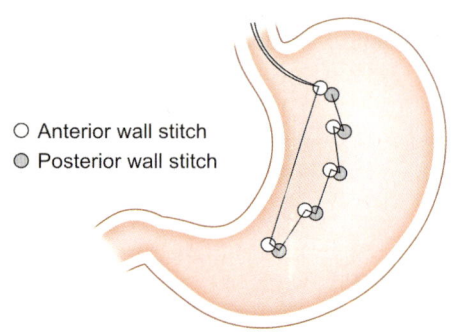

○ Anterior wall stitch
◉ Posterior wall stitch

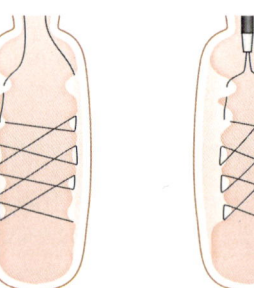

Balloon —

Fig. 21.6: Intragastric balloons

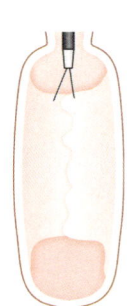

Fig. 21.7: Depicting transoral gastroplasty

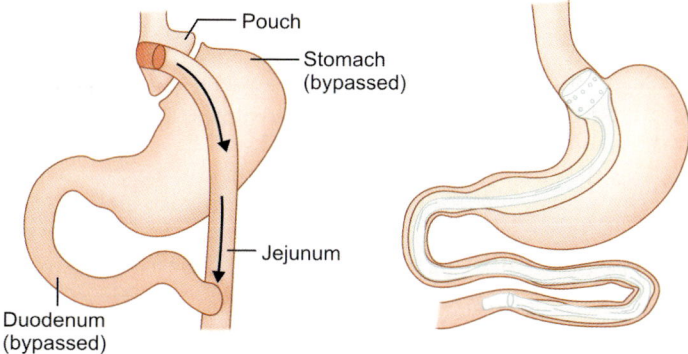

Fig. 21.8: Endoscopic duodenal jejunal sleeve

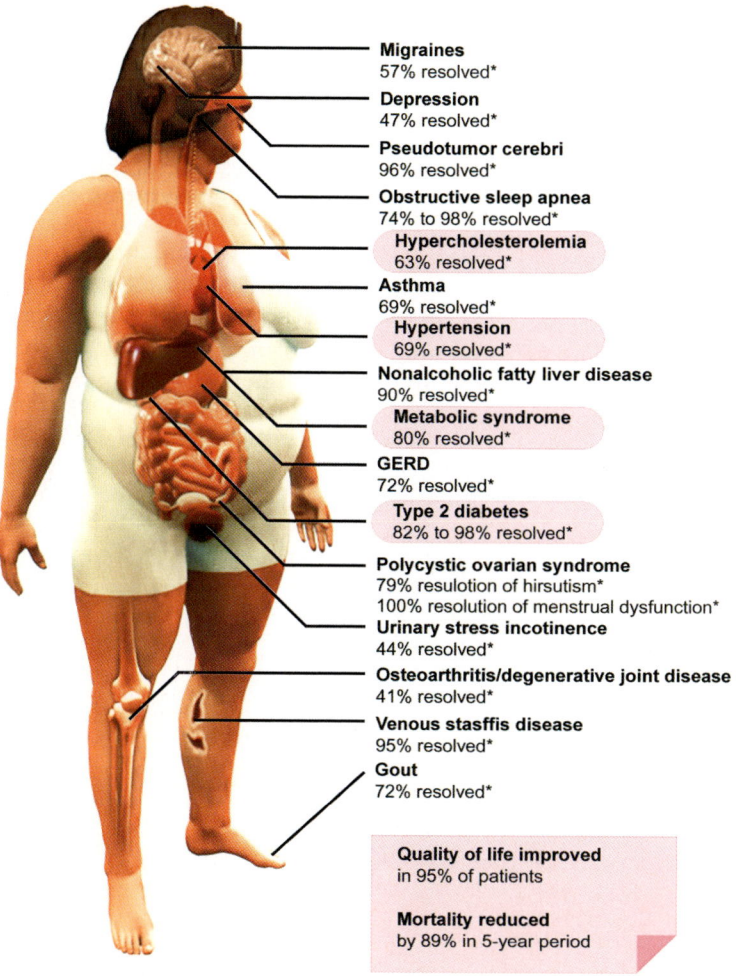

Migraines
57% resolved*

Depression
47% resolved*

Pseudotumor cerebri
96% resolved*

Obstructive sleep apnea
74% to 98% resolved*

Hypercholesterolemia
63% resolved*

Asthma
69% resolved*

Hypertension
69% resolved*

Nonalcoholic fatty liver disease
90% resolved*

Metabolic syndrome
80% resolved*

GERD
72% resolved*

Type 2 diabetes
82% to 98% resolved*

Polycystic ovarian syndrome
79% resulotion of hirsutism*
100% resolution of menstrual dysfunction*

Urinary stress incotinence
44% resolved*

Osteoarthritis/degenerative joint disease
41% resolved*

Venous stasffis disease
95% resolved*

Gout
72% resolved*

Quality of life improved
in 95% of patients

Mortality reduced
by 89% in 5-year period

Fig. 21.9: Benefits of the bariatric surgery/weight-loss surgery

Endoscopic Duodenal Jejunal Sleeve

It involves the implantation of a duodenal-jejunal bypass liner between the beginning of the duodenum and the mid-jejunum. This prevents the partially digested food from entering the first and initial parts of the small intestine, mimicking the effects of the bilio-pancreatic portion of Roux En-Y gastric bypass (RYGB) surgery (Fig. 21.8).

SUMMARY

If we consider bariatric surgery procedures in case of PCOS patients, it will not only improve the morbidities associated with the obesity but as weight reduction occurs it will be helpful in the ovulation as well as it will decrease percentages of the infertility (Fig. 21.9).

REFERENCES

1. Barham K. Abu Dayyeh, Elizabeth Rajan Christopher J. Gostout. Endoscopic Sleeve Gastroplasty a Potential alternative to surgical sleeve gastrectomy for treatment of obesity Gastrointestinal Endoscopy vol 78 issue 3 Sep 2013.

2. Butterworth J, Deguara J, Borg C-M. Bariatric Surgery, Polycystic Ovary Syndrome, and Infertility. Journal of Obesity. 2016

3. Shaveta M Malik, Michael L Traub. Defining the role of bariatric surgery in polycystic ovarian syndrome patients. World J Diabetes. 2012 Apr 15; 3(4):71–9.

4. Garruti G, Depalo R, Vita MG, Lorusso F, Giampetruzzi F, Damato AB, Giorgino F. Adipose tissue, metabolic syndrome and polycystic ovary syndrome: from pathophysiology to treatment. Reprod Biomed Online. 2009;19:552–63.

5. Teede HJ, Hutchison S, Zoungas S, Meyer C. Insulin resistance, the metabolic syndrome, diabetes, and cardiovascular disease risk in women with PCOS. Endocrine. 2006;30:45–53.

6. Diamanti-Kandarakis E. Insulin resistance in PCOS. Endocrine. 2006;30:13–7.

7. Essah PA, Wickham EP, Nestler JE. The metabolic syndrome in polycystic ovary syndrome. Clin Obstet Gynecol. 2007;50:205–25.

8. Cussons AJ, Stuckey BG, Watts GF. Metabolic syndrome and cardiometabolic risk in PCOS. Curr Diab Rep. 2007;7:66–73.

9. Traub ML. Assessing and treating insulin resistance in women with polycystic ovarian syndrome. World J Diabetes. 2011;2:33–40.

10. Moran LJ, Misso ML, Wild RA, Norman RJ. Impaired glucose tolerance, type 2 diabetes and metabolic syndrome in polycystic ovary syndrome: a systematic review and meta-analysis. Hum Reprod Update. 2010;16:347–63.

11. McCullough AJ. Epidemiology of the metabolic syndrome in the USA. J Dig Dis. 2011;12:333–40.

12. Ercan, C. et al M1363 Weight Reduction by means of an intragastric balloon in daily routine practise: Results at removal and in long term. Gastroentrol. 2010. 138(1):389.

13. Sarkhosh K, Sothilingam N,Switzer N, Karmali S. Emerging Techniques in Bariatric Surgery. The Fundamentals of Bariatric Surgery, Chapter 12.

Index

590